Eat To Beat
Disease Cookbook

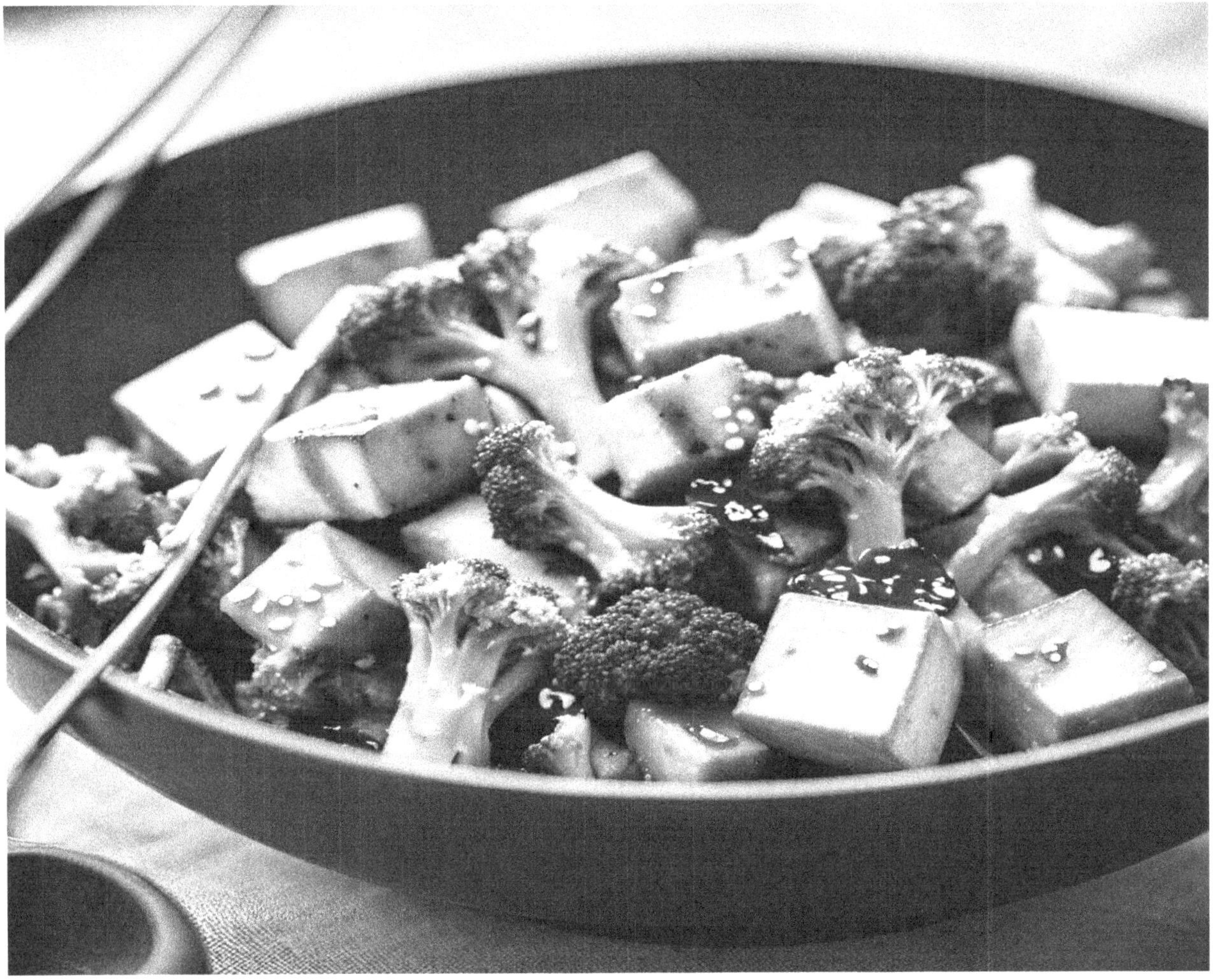

Harnessing the Healing Power of Food for Optimal Health

Monalisa Blake

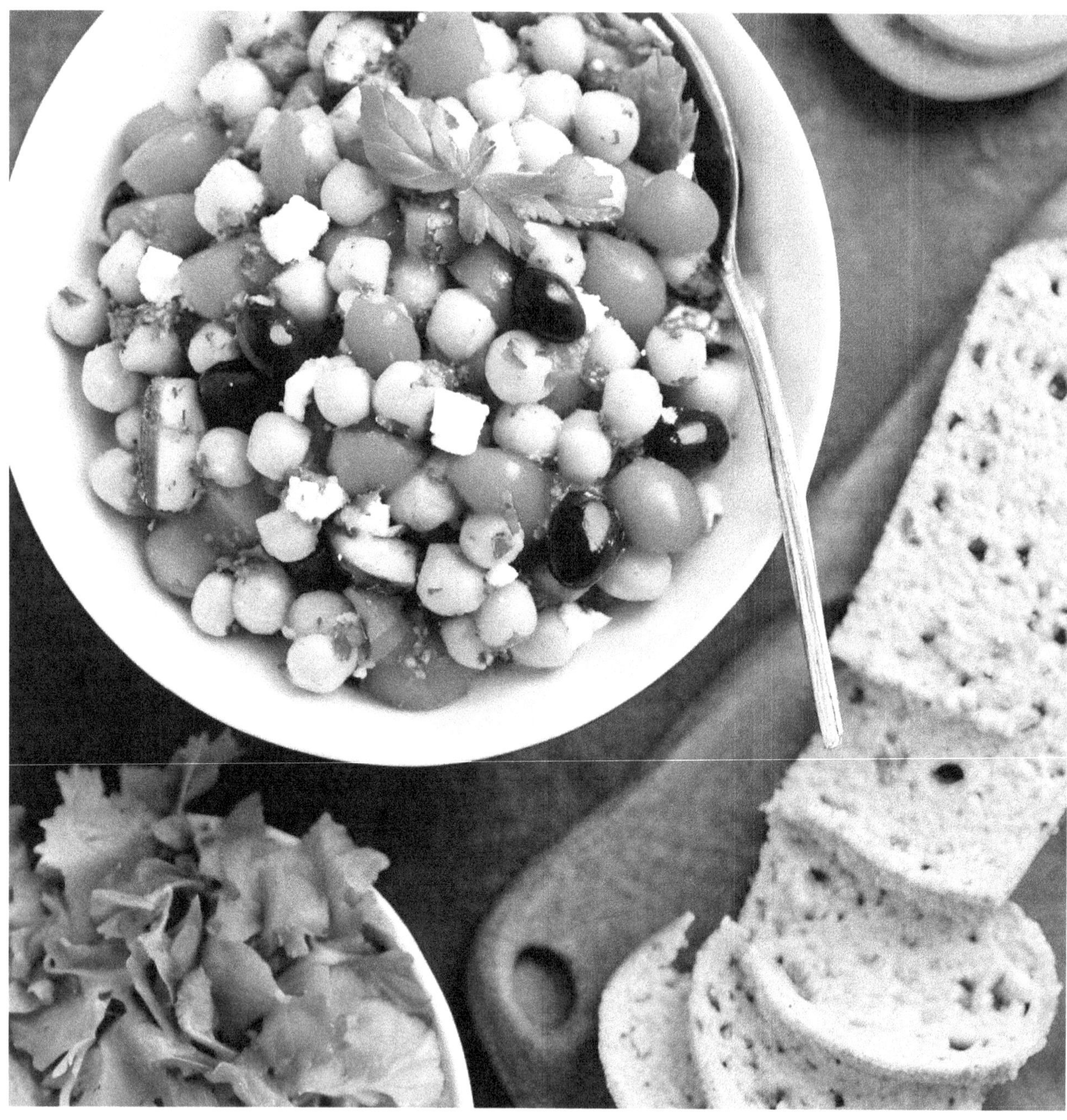

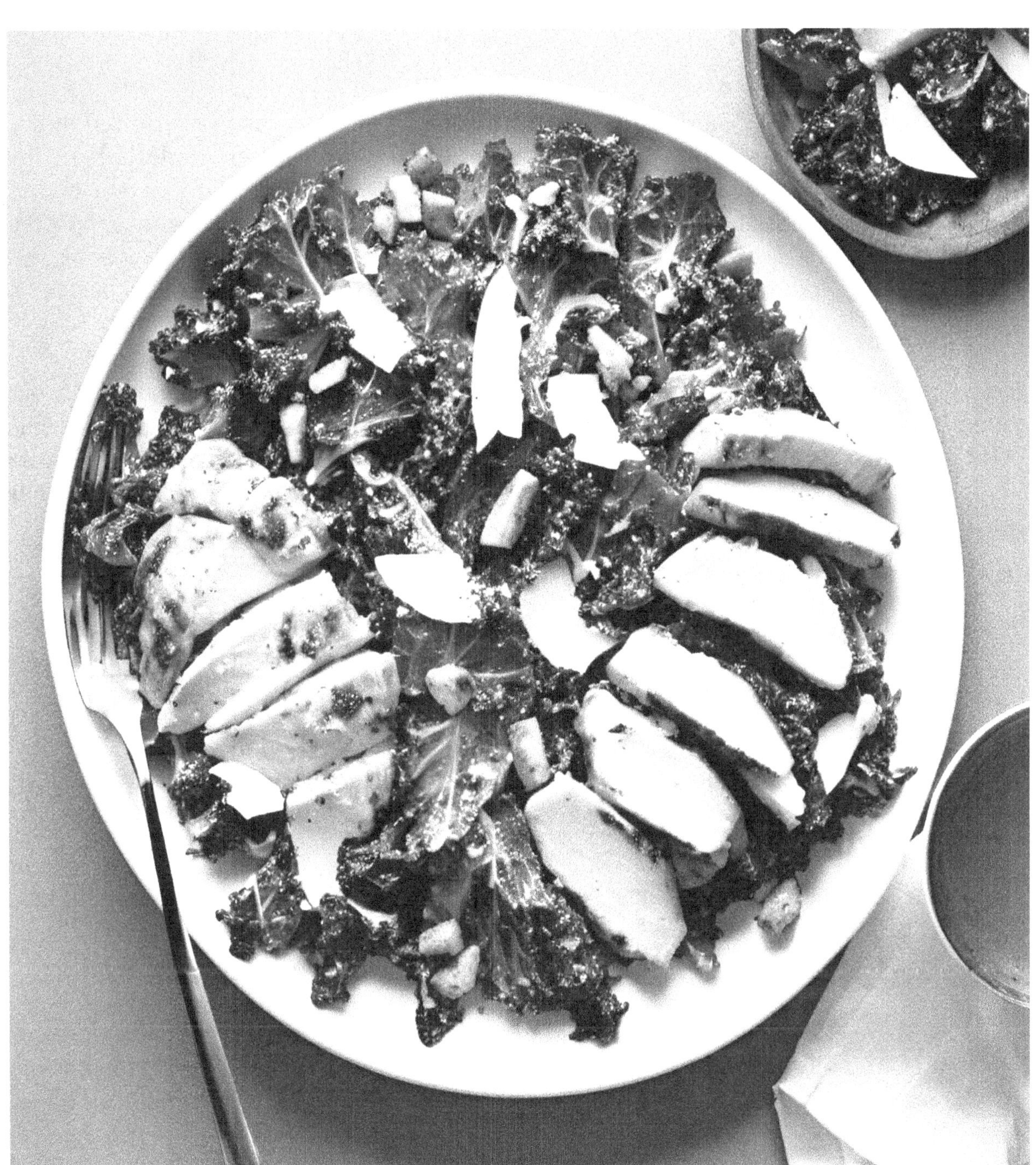

INTRODUCTION

Welcome to "Eat to Beat Disease: The Cookbook," a culinary journey inspired by the groundbreaking research that I have dedicated my career to exploring. In my previous work, "Eat to Beat Disease," I delved deep into the science of how our bodies possess incredible, innate defense mechanisms that can be activated and supported through the foods we eat. This cookbook is an extension of that research, offering you practical, delicious ways to incorporate health-promoting foods into your daily life.

The Power of Food as Medicine

The concept of food as medicine is not new, but modern science has given us a deeper understanding of how specific foods can influence our health at the molecular level. The foods we choose to consume can either support our body's defense systems or hinder them. By making informed choices, we can harness the power of food to enhance our health and well-being.

Chronic Disease Management

1. **Heart Health**: Incorporating heart-healthy foods such as fruits, vegetables, whole grains, and fatty fish rich in omega-3 fatty acids can lower blood pressure, reduce cholesterol levels, and decrease the risk of cardiovascular events.

2. **Diabetes Control**: Consuming low-glycemic index foods, fiber-rich whole grains, and lean proteins helps regulate blood sugar levels and may reduce the need for diabetes medications.

3. **Weight Management**: Choosing nutrient-dense, low-calorie foods and practicing portion control can support weight loss efforts and improve metabolic health.

Inflammation Reduction

1. **Anti-inflammatory Foods**: Certain foods like berries, fatty fish, leafy greens, nuts, and olive oil possess anti-inflammatory properties, which can help alleviate symptoms of inflammatory conditions such as arthritis and inflammatory bowel disease.

2. **Phytonutrients**: Plant compounds such as flavonoids, carotenoids, and polyphenols found in colorful fruits and vegetables have been shown to combat inflammation and oxidative stress.

Immune System Support

1. **Vitamin-Rich Foods**: Consuming foods high in vitamins A, C, D, and E, as well as zinc and selenium, strengthens the immune system and enhances the body's ability to fight off infections.

2. **Probiotics**: Fermented foods like yogurt, kefir, and kimchi contain beneficial bacteria that promote a healthy gut microbiome, which is essential for immune function.

Gut Health Optimization

1. **Fiber-Rich Foods**: High-fiber foods like fruits, vegetables, whole grains, and legumes promote digestive health by supporting regular bowel movements and feeding beneficial gut bacteria.

2. **Prebiotics**: Foods rich in prebiotic fibers, such as garlic, onions, bananas, and asparagus, nourish gut bacteria and contribute to a diverse microbiome.

Mental Well-being Enhancement

1. **Brain-Boosting Nutrients**: Omega-3 fatty acids found in fatty fish, nuts, and seeds support cognitive function and may reduce the risk of depression and anxiety.

2. **Mood-Enhancing Foods**: Foods rich in tryptophan, such as turkey, eggs, and tofu, and those containing magnesium, such as leafy greens and dark chocolate, can help regulate mood and reduce stress.

Bone Health Promotion

1. **Calcium and Vitamin D**: Consuming calcium-rich foods like dairy products, leafy greens, and fortified foods, along with adequate vitamin D from sunlight exposure or supplementation, supports bone strength and density.

2. **Magnesium and Vitamin K**: Foods rich in magnesium (nuts, seeds, whole grains) and vitamin K (leafy greens, broccoli) play a role in bone metabolism and may reduce the risk of osteoporosis.

Cancer Prevention

1. **Antioxidant-Rich Foods**: Fruits, vegetables, herbs, and spices contain antioxidants that neutralize free radicals and reduce the risk of cellular damage and cancer development.

2. **Cruciferous Vegetables**: Broccoli, cauliflower, Brussels sprouts, and kale contain compounds that may help prevent certain types of cancer by inhibiting tumor growth and promoting detoxification.

How to Use This Cookbook

Using this cookbook effectively involves more than just following recipes. It's about understanding how the foods you eat can support your health goals and incorporating them into your daily routine. Here are some tips on how to make the most out of 'Eat to Beat Disease: The Cookbook':

1. **Familiarize Yourself with the Five Defense Systems**: Before diving into the recipes, take some time to understand the five defense systems outlined in the book: angiogenesis, regeneration, microbiome health, DNA protection, and immunity. Knowing how these systems work will help you choose recipes that align with your health needs.

2. **Identify Your Health Goals**: Consider what specific health goals you want to achieve. Are you looking to boost your immune system, support heart health, or improve digestion? Knowing your goals will help you select recipes that target those areas.

3. **Explore the Recipe Labels**: Each recipe in the cookbook is labeled with the defense systems it supports. Pay attention to these labels as you browse through the recipes. This will make it easier for you to choose dishes that align with your health goals.

4. **Experiment with Ingredients**: Don't be afraid to get creative with the recipes. Feel free to swap **Ingredients** or modify the dishes to suit your tastes and dietary preferences. You can also use the cookbook as inspiration to create your own nutrient-packed meals.

5. **Plan Your Meals**: Take advantage of the meal planning resources provided in the cookbook. Use the weekly meal planner and shopping list essentials to plan your meals for the week ahead. This will help you stay organized and ensure you have all the **Ingredients** you need on hand.

6. **Focus on Variety**: Aim to incorporate a wide variety of foods into your diet. This will ensure you're getting a diverse range of nutrients and phytochemicals that support overall health. Don't hesitate to try new **Ingredients** and recipes to keep things interesting.

7. **Listen to Your Body**: Pay attention to how your body responds to different foods. Everyone's nutritional needs are unique, so it's essential to tune in to your body's signals and adjust your diet accordingly. If certain foods don't agree with you, try alternatives that provide similar health benefits.

8. **Stay Consistent**: Incorporating healthy eating habits into your lifestyle is a journey, not a destination. Be patient with yourself and stay consistent with your efforts. Over time, small changes can lead to significant improvements in your health and well-being.

Chapter One:

5 HORSEMEN of a Defense Systems

1. Angiogenesis:

Angiogenesis is the physiological process through which new blood vessels form from pre-existing vessels. This process is crucial for growth, development, and healing, as it supplies oxygen and nutrients to tissues, removes waste products, and supports the immune system. Angiogenesis plays a vital role in both health and disease, making it a significant area of study in medical research.

The Role of Angiogenesis in Health

In a healthy body, angiogenesis is tightly regulated, ensuring that new blood vessels form when and where they are needed. This regulation is essential for:

1. **Wound Healing**: When tissue is damaged, angiogenesis facilitates the growth of new blood vessels to supply the injured area with nutrients and oxygen, promoting faster healing.

2. **Reproduction and Development**: Angiogenesis is crucial during periods of rapid growth, such as embryonic development and in the menstrual cycle where the endometrial lining regenerates each month.

3. **Physical Exercise**: During exercise, muscles require increased blood flow to meet their heightened oxygen and nutrient demands. Angiogenesis helps to develop new capillaries in muscle tissues, enhancing athletic performance and recovery.

Angiogenesis in Disease

While angiogenesis is beneficial in many contexts, its dysregulation can contribute to several diseases:

1. **Cancer**: Tumors can hijack the angiogenesis process to create their own blood supply, enabling them to grow and metastasize. This process is known as tumor angiogenesis.

2. **Age-Related Macular Degeneration (AMD)**: Abnormal blood vessel growth in the retina can lead to vision loss.

3. **Arthritis**: Excessive angiogenesis in joint tissues can contribute to inflammation and pain.

4. **Obesity**: Increased fat tissue requires its own blood supply, leading to angiogenesis which can exacerbate weight gain and metabolic issues.

Dietary Impact on Angiogenesis

Research indicates that certain foods contain compounds that can influence angiogenesis, either promoting or inhibiting the process, which is the foundation of the concept of "food as medicine."

1. **Foods that Inhibit Angiogenesis**:

    - **Berries**: Rich in antioxidants, they contain compounds that can help inhibit the growth of abnormal blood vessels.

    - **Green Tea**: Contains catechins, which have been shown to inhibit angiogenesis.

    - **Tomatoes**: High in lycopene, which has anti-angiogenic properties.

    - **Dark Chocolate**: Flavonoids in dark chocolate can inhibit angiogenesis.

2. **Foods that Promote Angiogenesis**:

    - **Oysters**: High in zinc, which is essential for angiogenesis and wound healing.

    - **Citrus Fruits**: Contain vitamin C, important for the production of collagen and the formation of new blood vessels.

    - **Cruciferous Vegetables**: Such as broccoli and Brussels sprouts, which contain compounds that support healthy blood vessel growth.

2. Regeneration

Regeneration is one of the five key defense systems in the human body, highlighting its remarkable ability to repair, renew, and rejuvenate tissues and cells. This process is vital for maintaining health, recovering from injuries, and ensuring the proper functioning of organs and tissues throughout our lives.

The Science of Regeneration

At its core, regeneration involves the replacement of damaged or dead cells with new, healthy ones. This process is driven by stem cells, which have the unique ability to differentiate into various cell types needed for repair and maintenance. For example, the liver has a high regenerative capacity, able to repair itself even after significant damage, while other tissues like the heart have limited regenerative abilities.

Factors Influencing Regeneration

Several factors influence the body's regenerative capabilities, including age, genetics, overall health, and diet. As we age, the efficiency of regenerative processes typically declines, making it crucial to support these systems through lifestyle choices.

Foods That Promote Regeneration

Certain foods can enhance the body's regenerative abilities by providing essential nutrients and compounds that support stem cell function and tissue repair:

- **Oysters**: Rich in zinc, which is vital for cell growth and repair.

- **Kiwi**: High in vitamin C, an antioxidant that protects cells from damage and supports collagen production.

- **Cruciferous Vegetables (e.g., broccoli, Brussels sprouts)**: Contain sulforaphane, which has been shown to stimulate stem cell activity and promote detoxification.

- **Nuts and Seeds**: Provide healthy fats and proteins that are essential for cell membrane repair and function.

3. Microbiome Health

Microbiome health refers to the balance and diversity of the trillions of microorganisms residing in our gut. These microorganisms, including bacteria, viruses, fungi, and other microbes, play a crucial role in digestion, immune function, and overall health. A healthy microbiome contributes to efficient nutrient absorption, protection against pathogens, and regulation of the immune system.

Key Functions of a Healthy Microbiome

1. **Digestion and Nutrient Absorption**: Beneficial gut bacteria help break down complex carbohydrates, fibers, and proteins into simpler forms that can be easily absorbed by the body. They also produce essential vitamins like B and K.

2. **Immune System Regulation**: The gut microbiome educates and modulates the immune system, helping it to distinguish between harmful pathogens and the body's own cells, reducing the risk of autoimmune diseases and allergies.

3. **Protection Against Pathogens**: Healthy gut bacteria compete with harmful microbes, preventing them from colonizing the gut. They also produce substances that inhibit pathogen growth.

4. **Mental Health**: The gut-brain axis describes the bidirectional communication between the gut microbiome and the brain. A balanced microbiome can positively influence mood, stress responses, and cognitive functions.

Factors Influencing Microbiome Health

- **Diet**: A diverse diet rich in fruits, vegetables, whole grains, and fermented foods supports a healthy microbiome. Foods like yogurt, kefir, sauerkraut, and kimchi are particularly beneficial as they contain probiotics.

- **Antibiotics and Medications**: Overuse of antibiotics can disrupt the microbiome balance by killing beneficial bacteria. Other medications can also affect gut health.

- **Lifestyle**: Stress, lack of sleep, and sedentary habits can negatively impact microbiome diversity.

Supporting a Healthy Microbiome

To maintain a healthy microbiome, focus on a fiber-rich diet, including prebiotics and probiotics. Prebiotics, found in foods like garlic, onions, and bananas, feed beneficial bacteria. Probiotics, found in fermented foods, introduce live beneficial bacteria into the gut. Limiting processed foods, sugar, and artificial additives can also support microbiome health.

Foods that promote a healthy gut microbiome:

- **Yogurt**: Contains probiotics that enhance gut health.

- **Sauerkraut**: Fermented cabbage rich in beneficial bacteria.

- **Kimchi**: Fermented vegetables that support microbiome diversity.

- **Garlic**: Prebiotic properties feed healthy gut bacteria.

- **Bananas**: Provide prebiotics that support gut health.

4. DNA Protection: Safeguarding Your Genetic Blueprint

DNA protection is a critical aspect of maintaining health and preventing diseases like cancer. Our DNA is constantly exposed to potential damage from environmental toxins, ultraviolet radiation, poor dietary choices, and oxidative stress. Protecting and repairing DNA helps prevent mutations that can lead to serious health conditions.

Certain foods contain compounds that enhance the body's natural ability to protect and repair DNA. Carotenoids in carrots, polyphenols in green tea, and antioxidants in pomegranates are examples of such compounds. These foods neutralize free radicals, reducing oxidative stress and protecting cellular integrity.

Moreover, foods rich in folate, such as leafy greens, support DNA synthesis and repair, ensuring proper cell division and function. Omega-3 fatty acids found in fish also play a role in maintaining DNA stability by reducing inflammation.

Regular consumption of these foods can bolster the body's defense mechanisms, promoting the repair of damaged DNA and enhancing overall genetic health. By integrating DNA-protective foods into your diet, you can proactively reduce the risk of genetic mutations and support long-term health and longevity.

Foods that protect and repair DNA:

- **Carrots**: Rich in beta-carotene, protect against DNA damage.
- **Citrus Fruits** (oranges, lemons): High in vitamin C, which helps repair DNA.
- **Pomegranates**: Antioxidants protect against oxidative stress.
- **Spinach**: Contains folate, essential for DNA repair.
- **Walnuts**: Provide polyphenols that protect DNA.

5. Immunity

Our immune system defends us against infections and diseases. A strong immune system is essential for overall health. Key immune-boosting foods include garlic, mushrooms, elderberries, and green tea. Garlic has antimicrobial properties that help fight off infections, while mushrooms enhance the production and activity of white blood cells, essential for combating pathogens. Elderberries are rich in antioxidants and vitamins that support immune health, and green tea contains catechins, which have been shown to improve immune responses.

The book underscores the importance of a balanced diet rich in these foods to maintain a healthy immune system lifestyle factors such as adequate sleep, regular exercise, and stress management, which are crucial for optimal immune function. By integrating these immune-boosting foods and habits into daily life, individuals can strengthen their immune system, reduce the risk of illness, and promote overall health. This comprehensive approach to immunity showcases the powerful connection between diet and the body's natural defense mechanisms.

Foods that boost the immune system:

- **Garlic**: Has antimicrobial properties that enhance immune defense.
- **Mushrooms**: Enhance white blood cell activity.
- **Elderberries**: Rich in antioxidants and vitamins that support immunity.
- **Green Tea**: Catechins improve immune response.
- **Citrus Fruits**: High in vitamin C, essential for immune function.

Incorporating These Foods into Your Diet

Here are some practical ways to incorporate these foods into your meals:

- **Breakfast**: Add berries to your oatmeal or yogurt, enjoy a green tea, and sprinkle nuts on your cereal.

- **Lunch**: Include a spinach and mushroom salad, a side of fermented vegetables like kimchi, and a citrus fruit for dessert.

- **Dinner**: Prepare a salmon dish with a side of broccoli, and use garlic and turmeric in your seasoning.

- **Snacks**: Have a handful of walnuts, a piece of dark chocolate, or a kiwi.

- **Beverages**: Drink green tea throughout the day and enjoy a turmeric latte.

The Role of Diet in Disease Prevention

The foods we eat every day can have a profound impact on our health. Diet-related chronic diseases such as heart disease, diabetes, and cancer are major causes of morbidity and mortality worldwide. However, many of these diseases can be prevented, managed, or even reversed by making healthier food choices.

Cardiovascular Diseases (CVDs)

1. **Heart Health**: Consuming a diet rich in fruits, vegetables, whole grains, and lean proteins while limiting saturated fats, trans fats, cholesterol, sodium, and added sugars can reduce the risk of heart disease.

2. **Omega-3 Fatty Acids**: Found in fatty fish like salmon and walnuts, omega-3 fatty acids are beneficial for heart health, reducing the risk of arrhythmias and atherosclerosis.

Diabetes

1. **Balanced Carbohydrates**: Choosing complex carbohydrates with a low glycemic index, such as whole grains, legumes, and non-starchy vegetables, helps manage blood sugar levels and reduces the risk of type 2 diabetes.

2. **Fiber-Rich Foods**: Fiber slows down the absorption of sugar and improves insulin sensitivity, found in foods like oats, beans, fruits, and vegetables.

Obesity

1. **Caloric Balance**: Maintaining a balance between calorie intake and expenditure is crucial for weight management. Emphasizing nutrient-dense foods and portion control helps prevent obesity.

2. **Physical Activity**: Coupled with a healthy diet, regular physical activity supports weight loss and weight maintenance.

Cancer

1. **Plant-Based Diet**: Diets high in fruits, vegetables, whole grains, and legumes are associated with a reduced risk of certain cancers due to their rich antioxidant and anti-inflammatory properties.

2. **Limiting Processed Meats**: Reducing consumption of processed meats and limiting intake of red meat can lower the risk of colorectal cancer.

Osteoporosis

1. **Calcium-Rich Foods**: Adequate calcium intake from sources like dairy products, leafy greens, and fortified foods supports bone health and reduces the risk of osteoporosis.

2. **Vitamin D**: Obtaining sufficient vitamin D from sunlight exposure, fortified foods, and supplements aids in calcium absorption and bone mineralization.

Neurological Disorders

1. **Omega-3 Fatty Acids**: Consumption of omega-3 fatty acids found in fish, flaxseeds, and walnuts may reduce the risk of neurodegenerative diseases like Alzheimer's.

2. **Antioxidant-Rich Foods**: Antioxidants from fruits, vegetables, nuts, and seeds protect against oxidative stress, which is implicated in neurological disorders.

Digestive Health

1. **Fiber and Probiotics**: High-fiber foods and probiotic-rich foods like yogurt, kefir, and fermented vegetables support gut health, reducing the risk of gastrointestinal diseases.

2. **Hydration**: Drinking an adequate amount of water maintains digestive regularity and prevents constipation.

Immune System Function

1. **Vitamins and Minerals**: Consuming a variety of nutrient-rich foods ensures adequate intake of vitamins A, C, D, E, and zinc, which are essential for immune function.

2. **Protein**: Protein-rich foods like lean meats, poultry, fish, legumes, and dairy products provide the building blocks for immune cells.

Mental Health

1. **Omega-3 Fatty Acids**: Omega-3s play a role in brain health and may reduce the risk of depression and anxiety disorders.

2. **Complex Carbohydrates**: Whole grains, fruits, and vegetables provide sustained energy and support mood stability.

How to Use This Cookbook

This cookbook is divided into several chapters, each focusing on different meals and dietary needs. Whether you are looking for a hearty breakfast to start your day, a light lunch, a satisfying dinner, or a healthy snack, you will find recipes that are both delicious and nutritious. Each recipe is labeled with the defense systems it supports, making it easy for you to choose meals that meet your specific health goals.

Here are a few tips to help you get the most out of this cookbook:

- **Plan Ahead**: Take some time each week to plan your meals and create a shopping list. This will help you ensure that you have all the **Ingredients** you need on hand and make it easier to stick to your healthy eating plan.

- **Experiment with Ingredients**: Don't be afraid to try new foods and **Ingredients**. Many of the recipes in this book include options and variations, so you can tailor them to your tastes and dietary preferences.

- **Listen to Your Body**: Pay attention to how your body responds to different foods. Everyone is unique, and what works well for one person may not work as well for another. Find the foods that make you feel your best and incorporate them into your diet regularly.

Essential Ingredients for Health

Throughout this cookbook, you will find recipes that incorporate a variety of health-promoting foods. Here are some of the key **Ingredients** you will encounter and the benefits they offer:

- **Berries**: Rich in antioxidants, berries help promote healthy angiogenesis and protect against oxidative stress.

- **Green Tea**: Known for its DNA-protective properties, green tea also boosts immunity and supports overall health.

- **Garlic**: A powerful immune booster, garlic has anti-inflammatory and antimicrobial properties.

- **Dark Chocolate**: High in antioxidants, dark chocolate supports healthy angiogenesis and provides a delicious treat.

- **Fermented Foods**: Foods like yogurt, sauerkraut, and kimchi are excellent for maintaining a healthy microbiome and improving digestion.

The Journey to Better Health

Adopting a diet that supports your body's natural defense systems is a journey, and it's one that is well worth taking. The recipes in this cookbook are designed to make this journey enjoyable and sustainable. They are easy to prepare, delicious, and packed with nutrients that support your health.

I encourage you to approach this journey with an open mind and a willingness to try new things. Healthy eating doesn't have to be restrictive or boring. With a little creativity and the right **Ingredients**, you can enjoy a wide variety of delicious foods that are also incredibly good for you.

Real-Life Success Stories

One of the most rewarding aspects of my work has been hearing from people who have transformed their health by changing their diet. These success stories are a testament to the power of food as medicine. In this cookbook, you will find testimonials and case studies from individuals who have experienced significant health improvements by following the dietary recommendations from "Eat to Beat Disease."

These stories are not only inspiring but also provide practical examples of how you can incorporate health-promoting foods into your own life. They demonstrate that it is possible to take control of your health and make positive changes, no matter where you are starting from.

A Final Word

Thank you for choosing "Eat to Beat Disease: The Cookbook." I am excited to share these recipes with you and to help you on your journey to better health. Remember, the choices you make every day about what to eat can have a profound impact on your health and well-being. By choosing foods that support your body's natural defenses, you are taking a proactive step towards a healthier, happier life.

I hope you enjoy the recipes in this book as much as I have enjoyed creating them. Here's to delicious meals and a healthier you!

Chapter Two:

Essential Ingredients for Health

In "Eat to Beat Disease," this cookbook emphasizes on the importance of incorporating specific health-promoting foods into our diet. These **Ingredients** not only provide essential nutrients but also support the body's natural defense systems, helping to prevent and combat disease. Below is a detailed look at some of the key **Ingredients** highlighted in his research, along with their health benefits.

Berries

Types: Blueberries, strawberries, raspberries, blackberries

Health Benefits:

- **Antioxidants**: Rich in antioxidants like anthocyanins, which combat oxidative stress and inflammation.
- **Angiogenesis**: Promote healthy blood vessel formation, supporting cardiovascular health.
- **Cognitive Function**: Improve brain health and cognitive function, potentially reducing the risk of neurodegenerative diseases.

Ways to Include: Add to smoothies, yogurt, oatmeal, or eat as a snack.

Dark Chocolate

Type: Dark chocolate with at least 70% cocoa content

Health Benefits:

- **Flavonoids**: Contains flavonoids that improve blood vessel function and have anti-inflammatory properties.
- **Heart Health**: Supports cardiovascular health by enhancing circulation and reducing blood pressure.
- **Mood Enhancement**: Contains compounds that can boost mood and overall well-being.

Ways to Include: Enjoy a small piece as a dessert or add cocoa powder to smoothies.

Types: Matcha, sencha, gyokuro

Health Benefits:

- **Catechins**: Rich in catechins, which have antioxidant and anti-inflammatory properties.
- **DNA Protection**: Protects against DNA damage and supports immune function.
- **Weight Management**: Aids in weight management by boosting metabolism.

Ways to Include: Drink as a hot beverage, iced tea, or add matcha powder to recipes.

Garlic

Forms: Fresh garlic, garlic powder, aged garlic extract

Health Benefits:

- **Allicin**: Contains allicin, which has antimicrobial and immune-boosting properties.
- **Heart Health**: Helps lower cholesterol and blood pressure, supporting cardiovascular health.
- **Anti-Inflammatory**: Reduces inflammation and oxidative stress.

Ways to Include: Use in cooking, add to sauces, dressings, or roast whole cloves.

Turmeric

Form: Fresh turmeric root, turmeric powder

Health Benefits:

- **Curcumin**: Contains curcumin, a powerful anti-inflammatory and antioxidant compound.
- **Joint Health**: Reduces symptoms of arthritis and supports joint health.
- **Cancer Prevention**: Inhibits the growth of certain cancer cells and supports overall cellular health.

Ways to Include: Add to curries, soups, smoothies, or make turmeric tea (golden milk).

Tomatoes

Forms: Fresh tomatoes, tomato paste, tomato sauce

Health Benefits:

- **Lycopene**: High in lycopene, an antioxidant that supports heart health and reduces cancer risk.

- **Skin Health**: Protects skin from UV damage and promotes overall skin health.

- **Bone Health**: Contains vitamins and minerals that support bone health.

Ways to Include: Use in salads, sauces, soups, and as a base for dishes.

Nuts and Seeds

Types: Almonds, walnuts, chia seeds, flaxseeds, sunflower seeds

Health Benefits:

- **Healthy Fats**: Provide omega-3 fatty acids and other healthy fats that support heart and brain health.

- **Fiber**: High in fiber, aiding in digestion and promoting a healthy microbiome.

- **Nutrient-Rich**: Packed with vitamins, minerals, and antioxidants that support overall health.

Ways to Include: Add to salads, yogurt, oatmeal, smoothies, or eat as a snack.

Cruciferous Vegetables

Types: Broccoli, Brussels sprouts, kale, cauliflower

Health Benefits:

- **Sulforaphane**: Contains sulforaphane, which supports detoxification and has anti-cancer properties.

- **Fiber**: High in fiber, promoting digestive health and a healthy microbiome.

- **Vitamin C**: Rich in vitamin C, boosting immune function and skin health.

Ways to Include: Steam, sauté, roast, or add to salads and stir-fries.

Citrus Fruits

Types: Oranges, lemons, limes, grapefruits

Health Benefits:

- **Vitamin C**: High in vitamin C, essential for immune function, skin health, and DNA protection.

- **Flavonoids**: Contains flavonoids that support heart health and reduce inflammation.

- **Hydration**: High water content aids in hydration and overall bodily functions.

Ways to Include: Eat fresh, juice, add to salads, or use in dressings and marinades.

Fermented Foods

Types: Yogurt, kefir, sauerkraut, kimchi, miso

Health Benefits:

- **Probiotics**: Rich in beneficial bacteria that support gut health and a balanced microbiome.

- **Digestion**: Improve digestion and nutrient absorption.

- **Immune Support**: Strengthen the immune system by promoting a healthy gut environment.

Chapter Three:

Breakfasts to Boost Your Day

Blueberry Almond Overnight Oats

Prep Time: 5 minutes | **Cook Time**: 0 minutes | **Per Serving**: 1 serving

Ingredients:

- 1/2 cup rolled oats
- 1/2 cup unsweetened almond milk
- 1/4 cup Greek yogurt
- 1 tablespoon chia seeds
- 1/2 cup fresh or frozen blueberries
- 1 tablespoon almond butter
- 1 tablespoon sliced almonds
- 1 teaspoon honey or maple syrup (optional)

Instructions:

1. In a mason jar or a bowl, combine rolled oats, almond milk, Greek yogurt, and chia seeds. Stir well.
2. Add blueberries and almond butter, mixing them in gently.
3. Cover the jar or bowl and refrigerate overnight, or for at least 4 hours.
4. In the morning, give the oats a good stir, top with sliced almonds and a drizzle of honey or maple syrup if desired.
5. Enjoy your nutritious and delicious Blueberry Almond Overnight Oats.

Nutritional Value (Approx.):

Calories: 350 | Protein: 12g | Fiber: 8g | Healthy Fats: 14g | Carbohydrates: 42g

Green Tea Smoothie Bowl

Prep Time: 10 minutes | **Cook Time**: 0 minutes | **Per Serving**: 1 serving

Ingredients:

- 1 banana, frozen
- 1/2 cup spinach leaves
- 1/2 avocado
- 1 teaspoon matcha green tea powder
- 1/2 cup unsweetened almond milk
- 1 tablespoon chia seeds
- Toppings: fresh berries, sliced kiwi, granola, coconut flakes

Instructions:

1. Combine frozen banana, spinach leaves, avocado, matcha green tea powder, almond milk, and chia seeds in a blender.
2. Blend until smooth and creamy.
3. Pour the smoothie into a bowl.
4. Top with fresh berries, sliced kiwi, granola, and coconut flakes.
5. Enjoy your nutritious and energizing Green Tea Smoothie Bowl.

Nutritional Value (Approx.):

Calories: 300 | Protein: 6g | Fiber: 10g | Healthy Fats: 15g | Carbohydrates: 38g

Apricot Energy Balls

Prep Time: 15 minutes | **Cook Time**: 0 minutes | **Per Serving**: 12 balls

Ingredients:

- 1 cup dried apricots
- 1/2 cup almonds
- 1/4 cup rolled oats
- 2 tablespoons chia seeds
- 1 tablespoon coconut oil
- 1 tablespoon honey or maple syrup
- 1/2 teaspoon vanilla extract

Instructions:

1. Place dried apricots, almonds, and rolled oats in a food processor. Pulse until finely chopped.

2. Add chia seeds, coconut oil, honey or maple syrup, and vanilla extract. Process until the mixture is well combined and sticky.

3. Roll the mixture into 12 balls.

4. Place the energy balls on a baking sheet lined with parchment paper and refrigerate for at least 30 minutes.

5. Store in an airtight container in the refrigerator.

6. Enjoy your healthy and convenient Apricot Energy Balls.

Nutritional Value (Approx.):

Calories: 100 per ball | Protein: 2g | Fiber: 3g | Healthy Fats: 5g | Carbohydrates: 12g

Cinnamon-Walnut Oat Bake

Prep Time: 10 minutes | **Cook Time**: 30 minutes | **Per Serving**: 6 **Servings**

Ingredients:

- 2 cups rolled oats
- 1/2 cup chopped walnuts
- 1 teaspoon ground cinnamon
- 1/2 teaspoon baking powder
- 1/4 teaspoon salt
- 1 cup unsweetened almond milk
- 1/2 cup unsweetened applesauce
- 1/4 cup maple syrup
- 2 eggs
- 1 teaspoon vanilla extract

Instructions:

1. Preheat the oven to 350°F (175°C). Grease a baking dish with a little coconut oil or cooking spray.
2. In a large bowl, combine rolled oats, chopped walnuts, ground cinnamon, baking powder, and salt.
3. In another bowl, whisk together almond milk, applesauce, maple syrup, eggs, and vanilla extract.
4. Pour the wet **Ingredients** into the dry **Ingredients** and mix until well combined.
5. Pour the mixture into the prepared baking dish and spread it evenly.
6. Bake for 30 minutes or until the top is golden brown and the oat bake is set.
7. Let it cool for a few minutes before cutting into squares.
8. Enjoy your delicious and hearty Cinnamon-Walnut Oat Bake.

Nutritional Value (Approx.):

Calories: 250 per serving | Protein: 6g | Fiber: 4g | Healthy Fats: 12g | Carbohydrates: 30g

Peaches and Cream Oatmeal

Prep Time: 5 minutes | **Cook Time**: 10 minutes | **Per Serving**: 1 serving

Ingredients:

- 1/2 cup rolled oats
- 1 cup unsweetened almond milk (or any milk of choice)
- 1 fresh peach, sliced (or 1/2 cup canned peaches in juice, drained)
- 1 tablespoon Greek yogurt
- 1 teaspoon honey or maple syrup
- 1/2 teaspoon vanilla extract
- A pinch of cinnamon

Instructions:

1. In a small saucepan, combine oats and almond milk. Bring to a boil over medium heat.
2. Reduce heat and simmer, stirring occasionally, until oats are tender and the mixture is creamy, about 5-7 minutes.
3. Stir in vanilla extract and cinnamon.
4. Pour the oatmeal into a bowl, top with sliced peaches, a dollop of Greek yogurt, and a drizzle of honey or maple syrup.
5. Enjoy your comforting and nutritious Peaches and Cream Oatmeal.

Nutritional Value (Approx.):

Calories: 300 | Protein: 8g | Fiber: 6g | Healthy Fats: 5g | Carbohydrates: 55g

Savory Vegetable Breakfast Skillet

Prep Time: 10 minutes | **Cook Time**: 20 minutes | **Per Serving**: 2 **Servings**

Ingredients:

- 1 tablespoon olive oil
- 1/2 onion, diced
- 1 bell pepper, diced
- 1 zucchini, diced
- 1 cup cherry tomatoes, halved
- 1 cup spinach leaves
- 2 cloves garlic, minced
- 4 large eggs
- Salt and pepper to taste
- Fresh parsley, chopped (optional)

Instructions:

1. Heat olive oil in a large skillet over medium heat.
2. Add onion and bell pepper, and sauté until softened, about 5 minutes.
3. Add zucchini and cherry tomatoes, and cook for another 5 minutes, stirring occasionally.
4. Stir in spinach leaves and garlic, cooking until spinach is wilted.
5. Create four small wells in the mixture and crack an egg into each well.
6. Cover the skillet and cook until eggs are done to your liking, about 5-7 minutes.
7. Season with salt and pepper and garnish with fresh parsley if desired.
8. Enjoy your hearty and flavorful Savory Vegetable Breakfast Skillet.

Nutritional Value (Approx.):

Calories: 250 per serving | Protein: 15g | Fiber: 5g | Healthy Fats: 15g | Carbohydrates: 15g

Fluffy Sourdough Pancakes

Prep Time: 10 minutes | **Cook Time**: 15 minutes | **Per Serving**: 4 Servings

Ingredients:

- 1 cup sourdough starter (discard or active)
- 1 cup all-purpose flour
- 1 cup unsweetened almond milk (or any milk of choice)
- 1 egg
- 2 tablespoons honey or maple syrup
- 1 teaspoon vanilla extract
- 1 teaspoon baking soda
- 1/2 teaspoon salt
- Butter or oil for cooking

Instructions:

1. In a large bowl, mix the sourdough starter, flour, and almond milk until combined.
2. Add the egg, honey or maple syrup, and vanilla extract, and mix well.
3. Stir in baking soda and salt until just combined.
4. Heat a skillet or griddle over medium heat and lightly grease with butter or oil.
5. Pour 1/4 cup of batter onto the skillet for each pancake.
6. Cook until bubbles form on the surface and the edges look set, then flip and cook until golden brown.
7. Serve with your favorite toppings such as fresh fruit, maple syrup, or yogurt.
8. Enjoy your delicious and fluffy Sourdough Pancakes.

Nutritional Value (Approx.):

Calories: 200 per serving | Protein: 6g | Fiber: 2g | Healthy Fats: 4g | Carbohydrates: 36g

Mushroom and Tofu Scramble

Prep Time: 10 minutes | **Cook Time**: 10 minutes | **Per Serving**: 2 **Servings**

Ingredients:

- 1 tablespoon olive oil
- 1/2 onion, diced
- 2 cloves garlic, minced
- 1 cup mushrooms, sliced
- 1 block (14 oz) firm tofu, drained and crumbled
- 1/2 teaspoon turmeric
- 1/2 teaspoon cumin
- Salt and pepper to taste
- 1 cup baby spinach leaves
- Fresh chives, chopped (optional)

Instructions:

1. Heat olive oil in a large skillet over medium heat.
2. Add onion and garlic, and sauté until softened, about 3-5 minutes.
3. Add mushrooms and cook until they release their moisture and become tender, about 5 minutes.
4. Add the crumbled tofu, turmeric, cumin, salt, and pepper. Stir to combine and cook for another 3-5 minutes, until heated through.
5. Stir in spinach leaves and cook until wilted.
6. Garnish with fresh chives if desired.
7. Enjoy your protein-packed and flavorful Mushroom and Tofu Scramble.

Nutritional Value (Approx.):

Calories: 200 per serving | Protein: 15g | Fiber: 5g | Healthy Fats: 10g | Carbohydrates: 12g

High-Protein Green Tea Smoothie

Prep Time: 5 minutes | **Cook Time**: 0 minutes | **Per Serving**: 1 serving

Ingredients:

- 1 banana, frozen
- 1/2 cup Greek yogurt
- 1 teaspoon matcha green tea powder
- 1 scoop vanilla protein powder
- 1 cup unsweetened almond milk
- 1 tablespoon chia seeds
- 1/2 cup spinach leaves
- Ice cubes (optional)

Instructions:

1. Combine the frozen banana, Greek yogurt, matcha green tea powder, vanilla protein powder, almond milk, chia seeds, and spinach leaves in a blender.
2. Blend until smooth and creamy.
3. Add ice cubes if desired and blend again.
4. Pour into a glass and enjoy your nutrient-rich High-Protein Green Tea Smoothie.

Nutritional Value (Approx.):

Calories: 350 | Protein: 25g | Fiber: 6g | Healthy Fats: 8g | Carbohydrates: 45g

Spinach and Mushroom Egg Muffins

Prep Time: 10 minutes | **Cook Time**: 20 minutes | **Per Serving**: 6 muffins

Ingredients:

- 6 large eggs
- 1/2 cup milk (dairy or plant-based)
- 1 cup fresh spinach, chopped
- 1/2 cup mushrooms, diced
- 1/4 cup shredded cheese (optional)
- Salt and pepper to taste
- Olive oil for greasing

Instructions:

1. Preheat the oven to 350°F (175°C). Grease a muffin tin with olive oil.
2. In a bowl, whisk together the eggs and milk until well combined.
3. Stir in the chopped spinach, diced mushrooms, shredded cheese (if using), salt, and pepper.
4. Pour the mixture evenly into the muffin tin.
5. Bake for 20 minutes, or until the egg muffins are set and slightly golden.
6. Let cool slightly before removing from the tin.
7. Enjoy your protein-packed Spinach and Mushroom Egg Muffins.

Nutritional Value (Approx.):

Calories: 100 per muffin | Protein: 7g | Fiber: 1g | Healthy Fats: 6g | Carbohydrates: 3g

Chia Seed Pudding with Pomegranate

Prep Time: 5 minutes | **Cook Time**: 0 minutes (Chill for 4 hours) | **Per Serving**: 2 Servings

Ingredients:

- 1/4 cup chia seeds
- 1 cup unsweetened almond milk (or any milk of choice)
- 1 tablespoon honey or maple syrup
- 1/2 teaspoon vanilla extract
- 1/2 cup pomegranate seeds

Instructions:

1. In a bowl or jar, mix the chia seeds, almond milk, honey or maple syrup, and vanilla extract.
2. Stir well to combine and let it sit for about 10 minutes, then stir again to prevent clumping.
3. Cover and refrigerate for at least 4 hours, or overnight, until the mixture has thickened.
4. Stir well before serving and top with pomegranate seeds.
5. Enjoy your nutritious and refreshing Chia Seed Pudding with Pomegranate.

Nutritional Value (Approx.):

Calories: 200 per serving | Protein: 5g | Fiber: 12g | Healthy Fats: 8g | Carbohydrates: 25g

Avocado Toast with Tomatoes and Basil

Prep Time: 10 minutes | **Cook Time**: 0 minutes | **Per Serving**: 1 serving

Ingredients:

- 1 ripe avocado
- 1 slice whole-grain bread, toasted
- 1/2 cup cherry tomatoes, halved
- Fresh basil leaves, chopped
- Salt and pepper to taste
- A drizzle of extra-virgin olive oil

Instructions:

1. In a small bowl, mash the ripe avocado with a fork until smooth.
2. Spread the mashed avocado evenly on the toasted whole-grain bread.
3. Top with halved cherry tomatoes and chopped basil leaves.
4. Season with salt and pepper to taste and drizzle with a little extra-virgin olive oil.
5. Enjoy your delicious and healthy Avocado Toast with Tomatoes and Basil.

Nutritional Value (Approx.):

Calories: 300 | Protein: 5g | Fiber: 10g | Healthy Fats: 22g | Carbohydrates: 25g

Chapter Four:

Energizing Lunches

Quinoa and Broccoli Salad with Citrus Dressing

Prep Time: 15 minutes | **Cook Time:** 15 minutes | **Per Serving:** 4 servings

Ingredients:

- 1 cup quinoa, rinsed
- 2 cups water
- 1 head broccoli, cut into small florets
- 1 red bell pepper, chopped
- 1/4 cup red onion, finely chopped
- 1/4 cup toasted almonds, sliced
- 1/4 cup dried cranberries

Citrus Dressing:

- 1/4 cup olive oil
- 2 tablespoons fresh orange juice
- 1 tablespoon lemon juice
- 1 teaspoon Dijon mustard
- 1 teaspoon honey
- Salt and pepper to taste

Instructions:

1. In a medium saucepan, bring the quinoa and water to a boil. Reduce heat, cover, and simmer for 15 minutes or until the quinoa is cooked.
2. Meanwhile, steam the broccoli florets until tender, about 5 minutes.
3. In a large bowl, combine the cooked quinoa, steamed broccoli, red bell pepper, red onion, toasted almonds, and dried cranberries.
4. In a small bowl, whisk together the olive oil, orange juice, lemon juice, Dijon mustard, honey, salt, and pepper to make the dressing.
5. Pour the dressing over the salad and toss to combine.

6. Serve immediately or chill in the refrigerator for an hour for flavors to meld.

Nutritional Value (Approx.): Calories: 300 | Protein: 8g | Fiber: 7g | Healthy Fats: 14g | Carbohydrates: 38g

Lentil and Mushroom Stew

Prep Time: 10 minutes | **Cook Time:** 35 minutes | **Per Serving:** 4 servings

Ingredients:

- 1 tablespoon olive oil
- 1 onion, chopped
- 3 cloves garlic, minced
- 2 cups mushrooms, sliced
- 1 cup dried green lentils, rinsed
- 4 cups vegetable broth
- 1 can (14 ounces) diced tomatoes
- 2 carrots, sliced
- 2 celery stalks, chopped
- 1 teaspoon dried thyme
- 1 teaspoon smoked paprika
- 1 bay leaf
- Salt and pepper to taste
- Fresh parsley, chopped, for garnish

Instructions:

1. Heat olive oil in a large pot over medium heat. Add the onion and garlic, sautéing until soft, about 5 minutes.

2. Add the mushrooms and cook until they release their moisture and start to brown, about 5-7 minutes.

3. Stir in the lentils, vegetable broth, diced tomatoes, carrots, celery, thyme, smoked paprika, and bay leaf. Bring to a boil.

4. Reduce heat, cover, and simmer for 25-30 minutes, or until the lentils and vegetables are tender.

5. Season with salt and pepper. Remove the bay leaf before serving.

6. Serve hot, garnished with fresh parsley.

Nutritional Value (Approx.): Calories: 280 | Protein: 14g | Fiber: 12g | Healthy Fats: 5g | Carbohydrates: 45g

Mediterranean Chickpea Salad

Prep Time: 15 minutes | **Cook Time:** 0 minutes | **Per Serving:** 4 servings

Ingredients:

- 1 can (15 ounces) chickpeas, drained and rinsed
- 1 cucumber, chopped
- 1 cup cherry tomatoes, halved
- 1/4 red onion, finely chopped
- 1/4 cup Kalamata olives, pitted and sliced
- 1/4 cup feta cheese, crumbled
- 2 tablespoons fresh parsley, chopped

Lemon-Oregano Dressing:

- 1/4 cup olive oil
- 2 tablespoons fresh lemon juice
- 1 teaspoon dried oregano
- 1 teaspoon Dijon mustard
- Salt and pepper to taste

Instructions:

1. In a large bowl, combine the chickpeas, cucumber, cherry tomatoes, red onion, olives, feta cheese, and parsley.

2. In a small bowl, whisk together the olive oil, lemon juice, oregano, Dijon mustard, salt, and pepper to make the dressing.

3. Pour the dressing over the salad and toss to combine.

4. Serve immediately or chill in the refrigerator for an hour for flavors to meld.

Nutritional Value (Approx.): Calories: 250 | Protein: 8g | Fiber: 6g | Healthy Fats: 16g | Carbohydrates: 22g

Grilled Chicken and Kale Caesar Salad

Prep Time: 15 minutes | **Cook Time:** 15 minutes | **Per Serving:** 4 servings

Ingredients:

- 2 boneless, skinless chicken breasts
- 1 tablespoon olive oil
- 1 teaspoon garlic powder
- Salt and pepper to taste
- 6 cups kale, chopped and stems removed
- 1/4 cup grated Parmesan cheese
- 1/4 cup croutons (optional)
- 1/4 cup Caesar dressing (store-bought or homemade)

Instructions:

1. Preheat the grill to medium-high heat.
2. Brush the chicken breasts with olive oil and season with garlic powder, salt, and pepper.
3. Grill the chicken for 6-7 minutes per side, or until fully cooked. Let it rest for a few minutes before slicing.
4. In a large bowl, massage the kale with a pinch of salt for 2-3 minutes until tender.
5. Add the Parmesan cheese and croutons (if using) to the kale.
6. Toss the salad with Caesar dressing.
7. Top with sliced grilled chicken and serve immediately.

Nutritional Value (Approx.): Calories: 350 | Protein: 30g | Fiber: 5g | Healthy Fats: 20g | Carbohydrates: 12g

Spicy Black Bean Soup

Prep Time: 10 minutes | **Cook Time:** 25 minutes | **Per Serving:** 4 servings

Ingredients:

- 1 tablespoon olive oil
- 1 onion, chopped
- 3 cloves garlic, minced
- 1 jalapeño, seeded and chopped
- 1 red bell pepper, chopped
- 1 teaspoon ground cumin
- 1 teaspoon chili powder
- 1/2 teaspoon smoked paprika
- 3 cups vegetable broth
- 2 cans (15 ounces each) black beans, drained and rinsed
- 1 can (14 ounces) diced tomatoes
- 1 lime, juiced
- Salt and pepper to taste
- Fresh cilantro, chopped, for garnish
- Optional toppings: avocado slices, sour cream, shredded cheese

Instructions:

1. Heat olive oil in a large pot over medium heat. Add the onion, garlic, and jalapeño, sautéing until soft, about 5 minutes.
2. Add the red bell pepper and cook for another 3-4 minutes.
3. Stir in the cumin, chili powder, and smoked paprika, cooking for 1 minute until fragrant.
4. Add the vegetable broth, black beans, and diced tomatoes. Bring to a boil.
5. Reduce heat and simmer for 15-20 minutes, or until the flavors meld.
6. Using an immersion blender, partially blend the soup to your desired consistency.
7. Stir in the lime juice and season with salt and pepper.

8. Serve hot, garnished with fresh cilantro and optional toppings.

Nutritional Value (Approx.): Calories: 250 | Protein: 12g | Fiber: 10g | Healthy Fats: 7g | Carbohydrates: 36g

Tomato-Basil White Bean and Quinoa Salad

Prep Time: 15 minutes | **Cook Time:** 15 minutes | **Per Serving:** 4 servings

Ingredients:

- 1 cup quinoa, rinsed
- 2 cups water
- 1 can (15 ounces) white beans, drained and rinsed
- 2 cups cherry tomatoes, halved
- 1/4 red onion, finely chopped
- 1/4 cup fresh basil leaves, chopped
- 1/4 cup olive oil
- 2 tablespoons balsamic vinegar
- 1 teaspoon Dijon mustard
- Salt and pepper to taste

Instructions:

1. In a medium saucepan, bring the quinoa and water to a boil. Reduce heat, cover, and simmer for 15 minutes or until the quinoa is cooked. Fluff with a fork and let cool.

2. In a large bowl, combine the cooked quinoa, white beans, cherry tomatoes, red onion, and fresh basil.

3. In a small bowl, whisk together the olive oil, balsamic vinegar, Dijon mustard, salt, and pepper to make the dressing.

4. Pour the dressing over the salad and toss to combine.

5. Serve immediately or chill in the refrigerator for an hour for flavors to meld.

Nutritional Value (Approx.): Calories: 300 | Protein: 10g | Fiber: 8g | Healthy Fats: 14g | Carbohydrates: 36g

Waldorf Chicken Salad

Prep Time: 20 minutes | **Cook Time:** 0 minutes | **Per Serving:** 4 servings

Ingredients:

- 2 cups cooked chicken breast, diced
- 1 cup red grapes, halved
- 1 apple, cored and chopped
- 1 celery stalk, chopped
- 1/2 cup walnuts, toasted and chopped
- 1/4 cup Greek yogurt
- 1/4 cup mayonnaise
- 1 tablespoon lemon juice
- Salt and pepper to taste
- Fresh lettuce leaves, for serving

Instructions:

1. In a large bowl, combine the chicken, grapes, apple, celery, and walnuts.
2. In a small bowl, mix together the Greek yogurt, mayonnaise, lemon juice, salt, and pepper.
3. Pour the dressing over the chicken mixture and toss to combine.
4. Serve on a bed of fresh lettuce leaves.

Nutritional Value (Approx.): Calories: 350 | Protein: 26g | Fiber: 4g | Healthy Fats: 20g | Carbohydrates: 18g

Mediterranean-Style Tuna with Olives

Prep Time: 10 minutes | **Cook Time:** 0 minutes | **Per Serving:** 4 servings

Ingredients:

- 2 cans (5 ounces each) tuna in olive oil, drained
- 1/2 cup Kalamata olives, pitted and sliced
- 1/2 cup cherry tomatoes, halved
- 1/4 cup red onion, finely chopped
- 2 tablespoons capers, rinsed
- 2 tablespoons fresh parsley, chopped
- 2 tablespoons lemon juice
- 2 tablespoons olive oil
- Salt and pepper to taste

Instructions:

1. In a large bowl, combine the tuna, olives, cherry tomatoes, red onion, capers, and parsley.
2. In a small bowl, whisk together the lemon juice, olive oil, salt, and pepper.
3. Pour the dressing over the tuna mixture and toss to combine.
4. Serve immediately with whole-grain crackers or on a bed of greens.

Nutritional Value (Approx.): Calories: 250 | Protein: 22g | Fiber: 2g | Healthy Fats: 16g | Carbohydrates: 6g

Creamy Mushroom Soup

Prep Time: 10 minutes | **Cook Time:** 25 minutes | **Per Serving:** 4 servings

Ingredients:

- 2 tablespoons olive oil
- 1 onion, chopped
- 3 cloves garlic, minced
- 16 ounces mushrooms, sliced
- 1 teaspoon dried thyme
- 4 cups vegetable broth
- 1 cup unsweetened almond milk
- 1 tablespoon cornstarch mixed with 2 tablespoons water (optional, for thickening)
- Salt and pepper to taste
- Fresh parsley, chopped, for garnish

Instructions:

1. Heat olive oil in a large pot over medium heat. Add the onion and garlic, sautéing until soft, about 5 minutes.
2. Add the mushrooms and cook until they release their moisture and start to brown, about 8-10 minutes.
3. Stir in the dried thyme and cook for another minute.
4. Add the vegetable broth and bring to a boil. Reduce heat and simmer for 10 minutes.
5. Stir in the almond milk. If a thicker consistency is desired, add the cornstarch mixture and cook for a few more minutes until the soup thickens.
6. Season with salt and pepper.
7. Serve hot, garnished with fresh parsley.

Nutritional Value (Approx.): Calories: 180 | Protein: 6g | Fiber: 4g | Healthy Fats: 9g | Carbohydrates: 20g

Eggplant Salad with Walnuts and Mint

Prep Time: 15 minutes | **Cook Time:** 20 minutes | **Per Serving:** 4 servings

Ingredients:

- 1 large eggplant, cut into cubes
- 2 tablespoons olive oil
- Salt and pepper to taste
- 1/2 cup walnuts, toasted and chopped
- 1/4 cup fresh mint leaves, chopped
- 1/4 red onion, finely chopped
- 2 tablespoons lemon juice
- 1 tablespoon pomegranate molasses (optional)
- 1 tablespoon extra virgin olive oil

Instructions:

1. Preheat the oven to 400°F (200°C).
2. Toss the eggplant cubes with olive oil, salt, and pepper. Spread on a baking sheet and roast for 20 minutes, or until tender and golden brown.
3. In a large bowl, combine the roasted eggplant, walnuts, mint, and red onion.
4. In a small bowl, whisk together the lemon juice, pomegranate molasses (if using), and extra virgin olive oil.
5. Pour the dressing over the eggplant mixture and toss to combine.
6. Serve warm or at room temperature.

Nutritional Value (Approx.): Calories: 220 | Protein: 4g | Fiber: 6g | Healthy Fats: 16g | Carbohydrates: 18g

Kale Caesar with Parmigiano-Reggiano and Homemade Croutons

Prep Time: 15 minutes | **Cook Time:** 10 minutes | **Per Serving:** 4 servings

Ingredients:

- 6 cups kale, chopped and stems removed
- 1/4 cup Parmigiano-Reggiano, grated
- 2 cups bread cubes (day-old bread works well)
- 2 tablespoons olive oil
- Salt and pepper to taste

Caesar Dressing:

- 1/4 cup Greek yogurt
- 1/4 cup mayonnaise
- 2 tablespoons lemon juice
- 1 tablespoon Dijon mustard
- 1 teaspoon Worcestershire sauce
- 2 cloves garlic, minced
- Salt and pepper to taste

Instructions:

1. Preheat the oven to 375°F (190°C).
2. Toss the bread cubes with olive oil, salt, and pepper. Spread on a baking sheet and bake for 10 minutes, or until golden and crispy.
3. In a large bowl, massage the kale with a pinch of salt for 2-3 minutes until tender.
4. In a small bowl, whisk together the Greek yogurt, mayonnaise, lemon juice, Dijon mustard, Worcestershire sauce, garlic, salt, and pepper to make the dressing.
5. Toss the kale with the Caesar dressing and grated Parmigiano-Reggiano.
6. Top with homemade croutons and serve immediately.

Nutritional Value (Approx.): Calories: 280 | Protein: 8g | Fiber: 4g | Healthy Fats: 18g | Carbohydrates: 22g

Stone Fruit Salad with Honey Vinaigrette

Prep Time: 15 minutes | **Cook Time:** 0 minutes | **Per Serving:** 4 servings

Ingredients:

- 2 peaches, sliced
- 2 plums, sliced
- 2 nectarines, sliced
- 1/4 cup fresh basil leaves, chopped
- 1/4 cup goat cheese, crumbled (optional)
- 1/4 cup toasted almonds, sliced

Honey Vinaigrette:

- 2 tablespoons honey
- 2 tablespoons apple cider vinegar
- 1/4 cup olive oil
- Salt and pepper to taste

Instructions:

1. In a large bowl, combine the peaches, plums, nectarines, basil, goat cheese (if using), and toasted almonds.
2. In a small bowl, whisk together the honey, apple cider vinegar, olive oil, salt, and pepper to make the vinaigrette.
3. Pour the honey vinaigrette over the fruit mixture and toss gently to combine.
4. Serve immediately.

Nutritional Value (Approx.): Calories: 210 | Protein: 4g | Fiber: 4g | Healthy Fats: 14g | Carbohydrates: 20g

Chapter Five:

Healing Dinners

Garlic and Herb Baked Salmon

Prep Time: 10 minutes | **Cook Time:** 20 minutes | **Per Serving:** 4 servings

Ingredients:

- 4 salmon fillets (about 6 ounces each)
- 2 tablespoons olive oil
- 3 cloves garlic, minced
- 1 tablespoon fresh lemon juice
- 1 tablespoon fresh parsley, chopped
- 1 tablespoon fresh dill, chopped
- 1 teaspoon dried thyme
- Salt and pepper to taste
- Lemon wedges, for serving

Instructions:

1. Preheat the oven to 400°F (200°C).
2. In a small bowl, combine olive oil, minced garlic, lemon juice, parsley, dill, and thyme. Mix well to form a marinade.
3. Place the salmon fillets on a baking sheet lined with parchment paper.
4. Brush the marinade generously over each salmon fillet. Season with salt and pepper.
5. Bake in the preheated oven for 20 minutes, or until the salmon is cooked through and flakes easily with a fork.
6. Serve with lemon wedges on the side.

Nutritional Value (Approx.): Calories: 320 | Protein: 34g | Fiber: 0g | Healthy Fats: 20g | Carbohydrates: 2g

Spicy Turmeric Chicken with Sweet Potatoes

Prep Time: 15 minutes | **Cook Time:** 40 minutes | **Per Serving:** 4 servings

Ingredients:

- 4 boneless, skinless chicken breasts
- 2 tablespoons olive oil
- 2 teaspoons ground turmeric
- 1 teaspoon ground cumin
- 1 teaspoon smoked paprika
- 1/2 teaspoon cayenne pepper
- 3 cloves garlic, minced
- 2 large sweet potatoes, peeled and cut into 1-inch cubes
- Salt and pepper to taste
- Fresh cilantro, chopped, for garnish

Instructions:

1. Preheat the oven to 425°F (220°C).
2. In a small bowl, combine olive oil, turmeric, cumin, smoked paprika, cayenne pepper, and minced garlic to form a paste.
3. Rub the spice paste all over the chicken breasts.
4. Place the chicken and sweet potato cubes on a baking sheet lined with parchment paper.
5. Season with salt and pepper.
6. Roast in the preheated oven for 30-40 minutes, or until the chicken is cooked through and the sweet potatoes are tender.
7. Garnish with fresh cilantro before serving.

Nutritional Value (Approx.): Calories: 350 | Protein: 30g | Fiber: 5g | Healthy Fats: 12g | Carbohydrates: 30g

Mushroom and Barley Risotto

Prep Time: 15 minutes | **Cook Time:** 45 minutes | **Per Serving:** 4 servings

Ingredients:

- 1 cup pearl barley
- 2 tablespoons olive oil
- 1 onion, finely chopped
- 3 cloves garlic, minced
- 1 pound mixed mushrooms (such as cremini, shiitake, and button), sliced
- 1/2 cup dry white wine
- 4 cups vegetable broth, warmed
- 1/2 cup grated Parmesan cheese
- 2 tablespoons fresh parsley, chopped
- Salt and pepper to taste

Instructions:

1. Heat the olive oil in a large pan over medium heat.
2. Add the onion and garlic, cooking until soft and fragrant, about 5 minutes.
3. Stir in the mushrooms and cook until they release their juices and begin to brown, about 8 minutes.
4. Add the barley, stirring to coat in the oil, and cook for 2 minutes.
5. Pour in the white wine and cook until evaporated.
6. Gradually add the warm broth, one cup at a time, stirring frequently and allowing each addition to be absorbed before adding more.
7. Continue until the barley is tender and creamy, about 35 minutes.
8. Stir in the Parmesan cheese and fresh parsley, then season with salt and pepper to taste.

Nutritional Value (Approx.): Calories: 400 | Protein: 14g | Fiber: 8g | Healthy Fats: 14g | Carbohydrates: 52g

Mediterranean Stuffed Peppers

Prep Time: 20 minutes | **Cook Time:** 40 minutes | **Per Serving:** 4 servings

Ingredients:

- 4 large bell peppers (any color), tops cut off and seeds removed
- 1 cup cooked quinoa
- 1 can (15 ounces) chickpeas, drained and rinsed
- 1 cup cherry tomatoes, halved
- 1/2 cup Kalamata olives, sliced
- 1/4 cup red onion, finely chopped
- 1/4 cup fresh parsley, chopped
- 2 tablespoons olive oil
- 2 tablespoons lemon juice
- 1 teaspoon dried oregano
- Salt and pepper to taste
- Feta cheese, crumbled (optional)

Instructions:

1. Preheat the oven to 375°F (190°C).
2. In a large bowl, combine cooked quinoa, chickpeas, cherry tomatoes, olives, red onion, parsley, olive oil, lemon juice, oregano, salt, and pepper.
3. Stuff each bell pepper with the quinoa mixture and place them upright in a baking dish.
4. Cover the dish with foil and bake in the preheated oven for 30 minutes.
5. Remove the foil and bake for an additional 10 minutes, or until the peppers are tender.
6. Sprinkle with feta cheese, if using, before serving.

Nutritional Value (Approx.): Calories: 280 | Protein: 10g | Fiber: 8g | Healthy Fats: 12g | Carbohydrates: 36g

Tofu Stir-Fry with Ginger and Broccoli

Prep Time: 10 minutes | **Cook Time:** 15 minutes | **Per Serving:** 4 servings

Ingredients:

- 1 block (14 ounces) firm tofu, drained and cubed
- 2 tablespoons soy sauce
- 2 tablespoons olive oil, divided
- 2 cloves garlic, minced
- 1 tablespoon fresh ginger, grated
- 1 head broccoli, cut into florets
- 1 red bell pepper, sliced
- 1/4 cup vegetable broth
- 1 tablespoon cornstarch mixed with 2 tablespoons water (optional, for thickening)
- Sesame seeds, for garnish
- Cooked brown rice, for serving

Instructions:

1. In a bowl, toss the tofu cubes with soy sauce. Let it marinate for at least 10 minutes.
2. Heat 1 tablespoon of olive oil in a large skillet or wok over medium-high heat.
3. Add the marinated tofu and cook until golden brown, about 5-7 minutes. Remove and set aside.
4. In the same skillet, add the remaining olive oil, garlic, and ginger. Sauté for 1-2 minutes until fragrant.
5. Add the broccoli florets and red bell pepper slices, cooking for 5 minutes until tender-crisp.
6. Return the tofu to the skillet, add vegetable broth, and stir to combine.
7. If a thicker sauce is desired, add the cornstarch mixture and stir until the sauce thickens.
8. Serve hot, garnished with sesame seeds and accompanied by cooked brown rice.

Nutritional Value (Approx.): Calories: 250 | Protein: 14g | Fiber: 5g | Healthy Fats: 14g | Carbohydrates: 22g

Stuffed Bell Peppers with Quinoa and Spinach

Prep Time: 20 minutes | **Cook Time:** 40 minutes | **Per Serving:** 4 servings

Ingredients:

- 4 large bell peppers (any color), tops cut off and seeds removed
- 1 cup quinoa, rinsed
- 2 cups vegetable broth
- 2 tablespoons olive oil
- 1 small onion, finely chopped
- 3 cloves garlic, minced
- 2 cups fresh spinach, chopped
- 1 can (15 ounces) black beans, drained and rinsed
- 1/2 cup corn kernels (fresh or frozen)
- 1 teaspoon ground cumin
- 1/2 teaspoon smoked paprika
- Salt and pepper to taste
- 1/2 cup shredded cheese (optional)
- Fresh cilantro, chopped, for garnish

Instructions:

1. Preheat the oven to 375°F (190°C).
2. In a medium saucepan, bring the quinoa and vegetable broth to a boil. Reduce heat, cover, and simmer for 15 minutes, or until the quinoa is cooked.
3. In a large skillet, heat olive oil over medium heat. Add the onion and garlic, cooking until soft and fragrant, about 5 minutes.
4. Stir in the spinach, black beans, corn, cumin, and smoked paprika. Cook until the spinach is wilted, about 3 minutes. Season with salt and pepper.
5. Combine the cooked quinoa with the vegetable mixture.
6. Stuff each bell pepper with the quinoa mixture and place them upright in a baking dish.
7. Cover the dish with foil and bake in the preheated oven for 30 minutes.

8. Remove the foil, sprinkle with shredded cheese (if using), and bake for an additional 10 minutes, or until the peppers are tender and the cheese is melted.

9. Garnish with fresh cilantro before serving.

Nutritional Value (Approx.): Calories: 320 | Protein: 12g | Fiber: 10g | Healthy Fats: 12g | Carbohydrates: 44g

Ginger and Honey Glazed Tofu Stir-Fry

Prep Time: 10 minutes | **Cook Time:** 15 minutes | **Per Serving:** 4 servings

Ingredients:

- 1 block (14 ounces) firm tofu, drained and cubed

- 2 tablespoons soy sauce

- 1 tablespoon honey

- 1 tablespoon fresh ginger, grated

- 3 cloves garlic, minced

- 2 tablespoons olive oil, divided

- 1 head broccoli, cut into florets

- 1 red bell pepper, sliced

- 1/4 cup water or vegetable broth

- 1 tablespoon cornstarch mixed with 2 tablespoons water (optional, for thickening)

- Sesame seeds, for garnish

- Cooked brown rice, for serving

Instructions:

1. In a bowl, whisk together soy sauce, honey, ginger, and garlic.

2. Add the tofu cubes to the bowl, tossing to coat. Let it marinate for at least 10 minutes.

3. Heat 1 tablespoon of olive oil in a large skillet or wok over medium-high heat.

4. Add the marinated tofu and cook until golden brown, about 5-7 minutes. Remove and set aside.

5. In the same skillet, add the remaining olive oil and broccoli florets. Cook for 3 minutes.

6. Add the red bell pepper slices and continue to cook for another 3 minutes until vegetables are tender-crisp.

7. Return the tofu to the skillet, add water or vegetable broth, and stir to combine.

8. If a thicker sauce is desired, add the cornstarch mixture and stir until the sauce thickens.

9. Serve hot, garnished with sesame seeds and accompanied by cooked brown rice.

Nutritional Value (Approx.): Calories: 260 | Protein: 14g | Fiber: 4g | Healthy Fats: 14g | Carbohydrates: 24g

Tofu Stir-Fry with Ginger and Broccoli

Prep Time: 10 minutes | **Cook Time:** 15 minutes | **Per Serving:** 4 servings

Ingredients:

- 1 block (14 ounces) firm tofu, drained and cubed
- 2 tablespoons soy sauce
- 2 tablespoons olive oil, divided
- 2 cloves garlic, minced
- 1 tablespoon fresh ginger, grated
- 1 head broccoli, cut into florets
- 1 red bell pepper, sliced
- 1/4 cup vegetable broth
- 1 tablespoon cornstarch mixed with 2 tablespoons water (optional, for thickening)
- Sesame seeds, for garnish
- Cooked brown rice, for serving

Instructions:

1. In a bowl, toss the tofu cubes with soy sauce. Let it marinate for at least 10 minutes.

2. Heat 1 tablespoon of olive oil in a large skillet or wok over medium-high heat.

3. Add the marinated tofu and cook until golden brown, about 5-7 minutes. Remove and set aside.

4. In the same skillet, add the remaining olive oil, garlic, and ginger. Sauté for 1-2 minutes until fragrant.

5. Add the broccoli florets and red bell pepper slices, cooking for 5 minutes until tender-crisp.

6. Return the tofu to the skillet, add vegetable broth, and stir to combine.

7. If a thicker sauce is desired, add the cornstarch mixture and stir until the sauce thickens.

8. Serve hot, garnished with sesame seeds and accompanied by cooked brown rice.

Nutritional Value (Approx.): Calories: 250 | Protein: 14g | Fiber: 5g | Healthy Fats: 14g | Carbohydrates: 22g

Stuffed Bell Peppers with Quinoa and Spinach

Prep Time: 20 minutes | **Cook Time:** 40 minutes | **Per Serving:** 4 servings

Ingredients:

- 4 large bell peppers (any color), tops cut off and seeds removed
- 1 cup quinoa, rinsed
- 2 cups vegetable broth
- 2 tablespoons olive oil
- 1 small onion, finely chopped
- 3 cloves garlic, minced
- 2 cups fresh spinach, chopped
- 1 can (15 ounces) black beans, drained and rinsed
- 1/2 cup corn kernels (fresh or frozen)
- 1 teaspoon ground cumin
- 1/2 teaspoon smoked paprika
- Salt and pepper to taste
- 1/2 cup shredded cheese (optional)
- Fresh cilantro, chopped, for garnish

Instructions:

1. Preheat the oven to 375°F (190°C).

2. In a medium saucepan, bring the quinoa and vegetable broth to a boil. Reduce heat, cover, and simmer for 15 minutes, or until the quinoa is cooked.

3. In a large skillet, heat olive oil over medium heat. Add the onion and garlic, cooking until soft and fragrant, about 5 minutes.

4. Stir in the spinach, black beans, corn, cumin, and smoked paprika. Cook until the spinach is wilted, about 3 minutes. Season with salt and pepper.

5. Combine the cooked quinoa with the vegetable mixture.

6. Stuff each bell pepper with the quinoa mixture and place them upright in a baking dish.

7. Cover the dish with foil and bake in the preheated oven for 30 minutes.

8. Remove the foil, sprinkle with shredded cheese (if using), and bake for an additional 10 minutes, or until the peppers are tender and the cheese is melted.

9. Garnish with fresh cilantro before serving.

Nutritional Value (Approx.): Calories: 320 | Protein: 12g | Fiber: 10g | Healthy Fats: 12g | Carbohydrates: 44g

Ginger and Honey Glazed Tofu Stir-Fry

Prep Time: 10 minutes | **Cook Time:** 15 minutes | **Per Serving:** 4 servings

Ingredients:

- 1 block (14 ounces) firm tofu, drained and cubed
- 2 tablespoons soy sauce
- 1 tablespoon honey
- 1 tablespoon fresh ginger, grated
- 3 cloves garlic, minced
- 2 tablespoons olive oil, divided
- 1 head broccoli, cut into florets
- 1 red bell pepper, sliced
- 1/4 cup water or vegetable broth
- 1 tablespoon cornstarch mixed with 2 tablespoons water (optional, for thickening)
- Sesame seeds, for garnish
- Cooked brown rice, for serving

Instructions:

1. In a bowl, whisk together soy sauce, honey, ginger, and garlic.

2. Add the tofu cubes to the bowl, tossing to coat. Let it marinate for at least 10 minutes.

3. Heat 1 tablespoon of olive oil in a large skillet or wok over medium-high heat.

4. Add the marinated tofu and cook until golden brown, about 5-7 minutes. Remove and set aside.

5. In the same skillet, add the remaining olive oil and broccoli florets. Cook for 3 minutes.

6. Add the red bell pepper slices and continue to cook for another 3 minutes until vegetables are tender-crisp.

7. Return the tofu to the skillet, add water or vegetable broth, and stir to combine.

8. If a thicker sauce is desired, add the cornstarch mixture and stir until the sauce thickens.

9. Serve hot, garnished with sesame seeds and accompanied by cooked brown rice.

Nutritional Value (Approx.): Calories: 260 | Protein: 14g | Fiber: 4g | Healthy Fats: 14g | Carbohydrates: 24g

Elderberry and Beet Salad Kale and Pomegranate Salad Garlic Shrimp and Broccoli Stir-Fry

ChatGPT

Elderberry and Beet Salad

Prep Time: 15 minutes | **Cook Time:** 0 minutes | **Per Serving:** 4 servings

Ingredients:

- 4 medium beets, roasted and sliced
- 1/2 cup fresh elderberries (or 1/4 cup dried elderberries, rehydrated)
- 4 cups mixed greens (e.g., arugula, spinach, kale)
- 1/4 cup walnuts, toasted and chopped
- 1/4 cup feta cheese, crumbled (optional)
- 2 tablespoons olive oil
- 1 tablespoon balsamic vinegar
- 1 teaspoon honey
- Salt and pepper to taste

Instructions:

1. In a large bowl, combine the roasted beets, elderberries, and mixed greens.

2. In a small bowl, whisk together the olive oil, balsamic vinegar, honey, salt, and pepper.

3. Drizzle the dressing over the salad and toss gently to combine.

4. Top with toasted walnuts and feta cheese, if using.

5. Serve immediately.

Nutritional Value (Approx.): Calories: 180 | Protein: 4g | Fiber: 4g | Healthy Fats: 12g | Carbohydrates: 16g

Kale and Pomegranate Salad

Prep Time: 15 minutes | **Cook Time:** 0 minutes | **Per Serving:** 4 servings

Ingredients:

- 6 cups kale, chopped and stems removed
- 1 cup pomegranate seeds
- 1/4 cup sunflower seeds
- 1/4 cup goat cheese, crumbled (optional)
- 1/4 cup olive oil
- 2 tablespoons apple cider vinegar
- 1 tablespoon maple syrup
- Salt and pepper to taste

Instructions:

1. In a large bowl, massage the kale with a pinch of salt for 2-3 minutes until tender.

2. Add the pomegranate seeds, sunflower seeds, and goat cheese, if using.

3. In a small bowl, whisk together the olive oil, apple cider vinegar, maple syrup, salt, and pepper.

4. Drizzle the dressing over the salad and toss to combine.

5. Serve immediately.

Nutritional Value (Approx.): Calories: 220 | Protein: 6g | Fiber: 5g | Healthy Fats: 18g | Carbohydrates: 16g

Garlic Shrimp and Broccoli Stir-Fry

Prep Time: 10 minutes | **Cook Time:** 15 minutes | **Per Serving:** 4 servings

Ingredients:

- 1 pound large shrimp, peeled and deveined
- 1 head broccoli, cut into florets
- 3 cloves garlic, minced
- 2 tablespoons olive oil
- 1/4 cup low-sodium soy sauce
- 2 tablespoons honey
- 1 tablespoon rice vinegar
- 1 teaspoon fresh ginger, grated
- 1 tablespoon cornstarch mixed with 2 tablespoons water (optional, for thickening)
- Cooked brown rice, for serving

Instructions:

1. In a large skillet or wok, heat 1 tablespoon of olive oil over medium-high heat.
2. Add the shrimp and cook until pink and opaque, about 3-4 minutes. Remove from the skillet and set aside.
3. In the same skillet, add the remaining olive oil and garlic. Sauté for 1 minute until fragrant.
4. Add the broccoli florets and cook for 5 minutes until tender-crisp.
5. In a small bowl, whisk together soy sauce, honey, rice vinegar, and grated ginger.
6. Return the shrimp to the skillet and pour the sauce over the shrimp and broccoli. Stir to combine.
7. If a thicker sauce is desired, add the cornstarch mixture and stir until the sauce thickens.
8. Serve hot, accompanied by cooked brown rice.

Nutritional Value (Approx.): Calories: 260 | Protein: 25g | Fiber: 4g | Healthy Fats: 10g | Carbohydrates: 20g

Turmeric Chicken with Roasted Vegetables

Prep Time: 15 minutes | **Cook Time:** 40 minutes | **Per Serving:** 4 servings

Ingredients:

- 4 boneless, skinless chicken breasts
- 2 tablespoons olive oil
- 2 teaspoons ground turmeric
- 1 teaspoon ground cumin
- 1 teaspoon smoked paprika
- 1/2 teaspoon cayenne pepper
- 3 cloves garlic, minced
- 1 large sweet potato, peeled and cubed
- 2 carrots, sliced
- 1 red bell pepper, chopped
- Salt and pepper to taste
- Fresh cilantro, chopped, for garnish

Instructions:

1. Preheat the oven to 425°F (220°C).
2. In a small bowl, combine olive oil, turmeric, cumin, smoked paprika, cayenne pepper, and minced garlic to form a paste.
3. Rub the spice paste all over the chicken breasts.
4. Arrange the chicken and vegetables on a baking sheet lined with parchment paper.
5. Season with salt and pepper.
6. Roast in the preheated oven for 30-40 minutes, or until the chicken is cooked through and the vegetables are tender.
7. Garnish with fresh cilantro before serving.

Nutritional Value (Approx.): Calories: 350 | Protein: 30g | Fiber: 6g | Healthy Fats: 12g | Carbohydrates: 30g

Green Tea Poached Chicken with Brown Rice

Prep Time: 10 minutes | **Cook Time:** 25 minutes | **Per Serving:** 4 servings

Ingredients:

- 4 boneless, skinless chicken breasts
- 4 cups brewed green tea, cooled
- 1 tablespoon soy sauce
- 1 tablespoon honey
- 1 tablespoon fresh ginger, sliced
- 2 cloves garlic, crushed
- 2 cups cooked brown rice
- Steamed vegetables of your choice, for serving

Instructions:

1. In a large pot, combine brewed green tea, soy sauce, honey, ginger, and garlic. Bring to a simmer over medium heat.
2. Add the chicken breasts to the pot, ensuring they are fully submerged in the liquid.
3. Poach the chicken for 15-20 minutes, or until fully cooked.
4. Remove the chicken from the pot and let it rest for a few minutes before slicing.
5. Serve the poached chicken over cooked brown rice with steamed vegetables on the side.

Nutritional Value (Approx.): Calories: 300 | Protein: 28g | Fiber: 3g | Healthy Fats: 4g | Carbohydrates: 35g

Lentil and Sweet Potato Curry

Prep Time: 15 minutes | **Cook Time:** 30 minutes | **Per Serving:** 4 servings

Ingredients:

- 1 tablespoon olive oil
- 1 onion, chopped
- 3 cloves garlic, minced
- 1 tablespoon fresh ginger, grated
- 1 tablespoon curry powder
- 1 teaspoon ground turmeric
- 1/2 teaspoon ground cumin
- 1/2 teaspoon ground coriander
- 1 large sweet potato, peeled and cubed
- 1 cup dried lentils, rinsed
- 4 cups vegetable broth
- 1 can (14 ounces) coconut milk
- 1 can (14 ounces) diced tomatoes
- 2 cups fresh spinach
- Salt and pepper to taste
- Fresh cilantro, chopped, for garnish
- Cooked brown rice, for serving

Instructions:

1. Heat olive oil in a large pot over medium heat.
2. Add the onion, garlic, and ginger, cooking until the onion is soft and fragrant, about 5 minutes.
3. Stir in curry powder, turmeric, cumin, and coriander, cooking for another 1-2 minutes.
4. Add the sweet potato, lentils, vegetable broth, coconut milk, and diced tomatoes. Bring to a boil.

5. Reduce heat and simmer for 20-25 minutes, or until the lentils and sweet potato are tender.

6. Stir in the fresh spinach and cook until wilted, about 2 minutes. Season with salt and pepper.

7. Serve the curry over cooked brown rice, garnished with fresh cilantro.

Nutritional Value (Approx.): Calories: 400 | Protein: 14g | Fiber: 12g | Healthy Fats: 18g | Carbohydrates: 48g

Chapter Six:

Snacks and Desserts for Wellness

Dark Chocolate and Walnut Bites

Prep Time: 15 minutes | **Chill Time**: 1 hour | **Total Time**: 1 hour 15 minutes | **Servings**: 12 bites

Ingredients:

- 1 cup walnuts
- 1/4 cup dark chocolate chips
- 2 tablespoons honey
- 1/2 teaspoon vanilla extract
- Pinch of sea salt

Instructions:

1. In a food processor, pulse the walnuts until finely chopped.
2. Add the dark chocolate chips, honey, vanilla extract, and a pinch of sea salt to the food processor.
3. Pulse until the mixture comes together and forms a sticky dough.
4. Roll the mixture into small balls, about 1 tablespoon each, and place them on a baking sheet lined with parchment paper.
5. Chill in the refrigerator for at least 1 hour to set.
6. Once set, store the Dark Chocolate and Walnut Bites in an airtight container in the refrigerator for up to one week.
7. Enjoy these delicious and nutritious bites as a guilt-free treat!

Nutritional Value (Approx.): Calories: 90 | Protein: 2g | Fat: 7g | Carbohydrates: 7g | Fiber: 1g

Pomegranate Yogurt Parfait

Prep Time: 10 minutes | **Total Time**: 10 minutes | **Servings**: 1 parfait

Ingredients:

- 1/2 cup Greek yogurt
- 1/4 cup pomegranate seeds
- 2 tablespoons granola
- Drizzle of honey (optional)

Instructions:

1. In a serving glass or bowl, layer Greek yogurt, pomegranate seeds, and granola.
2. Repeat the layers until the glass or bowl is filled.
3. Drizzle with honey, if desired.
4. Serve immediately and enjoy this refreshing and nutritious Pomegranate Yogurt Parfait!

Nutritional Value (Approx.): Calories: 200 | Protein: 12g | Fat: 6g | Carbohydrates: 25g | Fiber: 3g

Turmeric Roasted Chickpeas

Prep Time: 5 minutes | **Cook Time**: 40 minutes | **Total Time**: 45 minutes | **Servings**: 4

Ingredients:

- 2 cans (15 ounces each) chickpeas, drained, rinsed, and patted dry
- 2 tablespoons olive oil
- 1 tablespoon ground turmeric
- 1 teaspoon ground cumin
- 1 teaspoon paprika
- 1/2 teaspoon garlic powder
- Salt to taste

Instructions:

1. Preheat the oven to 400°F (200°C) and line a baking sheet with parchment paper.
2. In a large mixing bowl, toss the chickpeas with olive oil, ground turmeric, ground cumin, paprika, garlic powder, and salt until evenly coated.
3. Spread the seasoned chickpeas in a single layer on the prepared baking sheet.
4. Bake in the preheated oven for 35-40 minutes, shaking the pan halfway through, until the chickpeas are crispy.
5. Remove from the oven and let them cool slightly before serving.
6. Enjoy these flavorful Turmeric Roasted Chickpeas as a crunchy and healthy snack!

Nutritional Value (Approx.): Calories: 220 | Protein: 8g | Fat: 8g | Carbohydrates: 30g | Fiber: 8g

Berry and Oatmeal Bars

Prep Time: 15 minutes | **Cook Time**: 25 minutes | **Total Time**: 40 minutes | **Servings**: 12 bars

Ingredients:

- 2 cups rolled oats
- 1 cup mixed berries (such as strawberries, blueberries, raspberries)
- 1/2 cup almond butter
- 1/4 cup honey
- 1/4 cup unsweetened applesauce
- 1 teaspoon vanilla extract
- 1/2 teaspoon ground cinnamon
- Pinch of salt

Instructions:

1. Preheat the oven to 350°F (175°C) and line an 8x8-inch baking dish with parchment paper, leaving some overhang on the sides.
2. In a large mixing bowl, combine rolled oats, mixed berries, almond butter, honey, applesauce, vanilla extract, ground cinnamon, and a pinch of salt. Mix until well combined.
3. Press the mixture evenly into the prepared baking dish.
4. Bake in the preheated oven for 25 30 minutes, or until the edges are golden brown.
5. Remove from the oven and let it cool completely in the baking dish.
6. Once cooled, lift the bars out of the baking dish using the parchment paper overhang and transfer to a cutting board.
7. Cut into bars using a sharp knife.
8. Store the bars in an airtight container for up to one week.
9. Enjoy these wholesome Berry and Oatmeal Bars as a nutritious snack or breakfast option!

Nutritional Value (Approx.): Calories: 150 | Protein: 4g | Fat: 7g | Carbohydrates: 20g | Fiber: 3g

Roasted Chickpeas with Spices

Prep Time: 10 minutes | **Cook Time**: 40 minutes | **Total Time**: 50 minutes | **Servings**: 4

Ingredients:

- 2 cans (15 ounces each) chickpeas, drained, rinsed, and patted dry
- 2 tablespoons olive oil
- 1 teaspoon ground cumin
- 1 teaspoon smoked paprika
- 1/2 teaspoon garlic powder
- 1/2 teaspoon onion powder
- 1/4 teaspoon cayenne pepper (optional)
- Salt to taste

Instructions:

1. Preheat the oven to 400°F (200°C) and line a baking sheet with parchment paper.
2. In a large mixing bowl, toss the chickpeas with olive oil, ground cumin, smoked paprika, garlic powder, onion powder, cayenne pepper (if using), and salt until evenly coated.
3. Spread the seasoned chickpeas in a single layer on the prepared baking sheet.
4. Bake in the preheated oven for 35-40 minutes, shaking the pan halfway through, until the chickpeas are golden brown and crispy.
5. Remove from the oven and let them cool slightly before serving.
6. Enjoy these flavorful Roasted Chickpeas with Spices as a crunchy snack or salad topper!

Nutritional Value (Approx.): Calories: 200 | Protein: 7g | Fat: 7g | Carbohydrates: 27g | Fiber: 7g

Matcha Green Tea Energy Balls

Prep Time: 10 minutes | **Chill Time**: 30 minutes | **Total Time**: 40 minutes | **Servings**: 12 balls

Ingredients:

- 1 cup rolled oats
- 1/2 cup almond butter
- 1/4 cup honey
- 2 tablespoons matcha green tea powder
- 1/4 cup shredded coconut (unsweetened)
- 1/4 cup dark chocolate chips

Instructions:

1. In a large mixing bowl, combine rolled oats, almond butter, honey, matcha green tea powder, shredded coconut, and dark chocolate chips.

2. Mix well until all Ingredients are evenly incorporated.

3. Using your hands, roll the mixture into 1-inch balls and place them on a baking sheet lined with parchment paper.

4. Once all the mixture is rolled into balls, transfer the baking sheet to the refrigerator and chill for at least 30 minutes to set.

5. Once chilled, store the Matcha Green Tea Energy Balls in an airtight container in the refrigerator for up to one week.

6. Enjoy these nutritious and energizing snacks whenever you need a quick boost of energy!

Nutritional Value (Approx.): Calories: 120 | Protein: 3g | Fat: 6g | Carbohydrates: 14g | Fiber: 2g

Pistachio Bars

Prep Time: 15 minutes | **Chill Time**: 2 hours | **Total Time**: 2 hours 15 minutes | **Servings**: 12 bars

Ingredients:

- 1 cup shelled pistachios
- 1 cup dates, pitted
- 1/4 cup dried cranberries
- 1/4 cup shredded coconut (unsweetened)
- 1 tablespoon honey
- 1/2 teaspoon vanilla extract
- Pinch of sea salt

Instructions:

1. In a food processor, pulse the shelled pistachios until finely chopped.
2. Add the pitted dates, dried cranberries, shredded coconut, honey, vanilla extract, and a pinch of sea salt to the food processor.
3. Process the mixture until it comes together into a sticky dough-like consistency.
4. Line a square baking dish with parchment paper, leaving some overhang on the sides for easy removal.
5. Transfer the mixture into the lined baking dish and press it evenly into the bottom using your hands or the back of a spoon.
6. Place the baking dish in the refrigerator and chill for at least 2 hours to firm up.
7. Once chilled and firm, remove the pistachio mixture from the baking dish using the parchment paper overhang.
8. Cut into bars using a sharp knife.
9. Store the Pistachio Bars in an airtight container in the refrigerator for up to one week.
10. Enjoy these delicious and nutrient-packed bars as a wholesome snack or dessert option!

Nutritional Value (Approx.): Calories: 150 | Protein: 4g | Fat: 7g | Carbohydrates: 20g | Fiber: 3g

Raspberry, Ginger, and Hazelnut Chia Pudding

Prep Time: 5 minutes | **Chill Time**: 4 hours | **Total Time**: 4 hours 5 minutes | **Servings**: 2

Ingredients:

- 1/2 cup fresh raspberries

- 2 tablespoons chia seeds

- 1 cup almond milk

- 1 tablespoon maple syrup (optional)

- 1 tablespoon chopped hazelnuts

- 1 teaspoon grated fresh ginger

- Dash of vanilla extract

Instructions:

1. In a mixing bowl, mash the raspberries using a fork.

2. Add chia seeds, almond milk, maple syrup (if using), chopped hazelnuts, grated fresh ginger, and vanilla extract to the mashed raspberries. Stir well to combine.

3. Cover the bowl and refrigerate for at least 4 hours or overnight, until the mixture thickens and sets into a pudding-like consistency.

4. Once chilled and set, stir the chia pudding to distribute the Ingredients evenly.

5. Divide the Raspberry, Ginger, and Hazelnut Chia Pudding into serving glasses or bowls.

6. Garnish with additional raspberries, hazelnuts, or a drizzle of maple syrup, if desired.

7. Enjoy this delicious and nutritious chia pudding as a satisfying breakfast or snack!

Nutritional Value (Approx.): Calories: 150 | Protein: 4g | Fat: 9g | Carbohydrates: 14g | Fiber: 8g

Spiced Carrot and Nut Muffins

Prep Time: 15 minutes | **Cook Time**: 20 minutes | **Total Time**: 35 minutes | **Servings**: 12 muffins

Ingredients:

- 1 1/2 cups whole wheat flour
- 1 teaspoon baking powder
- 1/2 teaspoon baking soda
- 1/2 teaspoon ground cinnamon
- 1/4 teaspoon ground nutmeg
- Pinch of salt
- 1/2 cup grated carrots
- 1/2 cup chopped nuts (walnuts, pecans, or almonds)
- 1/4 cup raisins or chopped dried fruits
- 1/4 cup maple syrup or honey
- 1/4 cup unsweetened applesauce
- 1/4 cup plain Greek yogurt
- 1/4 cup milk (dairy or plant-based)
- 1 egg
- 1 teaspoon vanilla extract

Instructions:

1. Preheat the oven to 375°F (190°C) and line a muffin tin with paper liners or grease the cups.

2. In a large mixing bowl, whisk together the whole wheat flour, baking powder, baking soda, ground cinnamon, ground nutmeg, and salt.

3. In a separate bowl, combine grated carrots, chopped nuts, raisins or dried fruits, maple syrup or honey, unsweetened applesauce, Greek yogurt, milk, egg, and vanilla extract. Mix until well combined.

4. Pour the wet Ingredients into the dry Ingredients and gently fold until just combined. Do not overmix.

5. Divide the batter evenly among the prepared muffin cups, filling each about 2/3 full.

6. Bake in the preheated oven for 18-20 minutes, or until a toothpick inserted into the center of a muffin comes out clean.

7. Remove from the oven and let the muffins cool in the tin for 5 minutes before transferring them to a wire rack to cool completely.

8. Once cooled, store the Spiced Carrot and Nut Muffins in an airtight container at room temperature for up to 3 days, or freeze for longer storage.

9. Enjoy these moist and flavorful muffins as a wholesome breakfast or snack!

Nutritional Value (Approx.): Calories: 150 | Protein: 4g | Fat: 6g | Carbohydrates: 22g | Fiber: 3g

Basic, No-Knead Sourdough Smoothie

Prep Time: 5 minutes | **Total Time**: 5 minutes | **Servings**: 1 smoothie

Ingredients:

- 1 cup fresh spinach leaves
- 1/2 cup diced ripe mango
- 1/2 cup diced ripe banana
- 1/2 cup plain Greek yogurt
- 1/4 cup no-knead sourdough starter discard
- 1/2 cup unsweetened almond milk or any milk of your choice
- 1 tablespoon honey or maple syrup (optional)
- Ice cubes (optional)

Instructions:

1. Place fresh spinach leaves, diced mango, diced banana, plain Greek yogurt, no-knead sourdough starter discard, almond milk, and honey or maple syrup (if using) in a blender.

2. Blend until smooth and creamy.

3. If desired, add ice cubes to the blender and blend again until smooth.

4. Pour the smoothie into a glass and serve immediately.

5. Enjoy this nutrient-rich Basic, No-Knead Sourdough Smoothie as a refreshing and healthy beverage!

Nutritional Value (Approx.): Calories: 250 | Protein: 12g | Fat: 4g | Carbohydrates: 45g | Fiber: 6g

Chapter Seven:

Drinks and Smoothies

Anti-Inflammatory Golden Milk

Prep Time: 5 minutes | **Cook Time**: 5 minutes | **Total Time**: 10 minutes | **Servings**: 1

Ingredients:

- 1 cup unsweetened almond milk (or any milk of your choice)
- 1 teaspoon ground turmeric
- 1/2 teaspoon ground cinnamon
- 1/4 teaspoon ground ginger
- Pinch of black pepper
- 1 teaspoon honey or maple syrup (optional)

Instructions:

1. In a small saucepan, heat the almond milk over medium heat until warmed but not boiling.
2. Stir in the ground turmeric, ground cinnamon, ground ginger, and a pinch of black pepper.
3. Continue to cook for 2-3 minutes, stirring constantly, until the spices are well incorporated and the mixture is heated through.
4. Remove from heat and sweeten with honey or maple syrup, if desired.
5. Pour the Anti-Inflammatory Golden Milk into a mug and enjoy it warm.
6. Feel free to adjust the sweetness and spices according to your taste preferences.
7. This soothing drink is perfect for relaxing evenings or as a comforting beverage any time of the day.

Nutritional Value (Approx.): Calories: 50 | Protein: 1g | Fat: 3g | Carbohydrates: 6g | Fiber: 1g

Berry and Beet Detox Smoothie

Prep Time: 5 minutes | **Total Time**: 5 minutes | **Servings**: 1

Ingredients:

- 1/2 cup mixed berries (such as strawberries, blueberries, raspberries)
- 1/2 small cooked beet, peeled and diced
- 1/2 cup plain Greek yogurt
- 1/2 cup unsweetened almond milk (or any milk of your choice)
- 1 tablespoon chia seeds
- 1 teaspoon honey or maple syrup (optional)
- Ice cubes (optional)

Instructions:

1. Place mixed berries, cooked beet, plain Greek yogurt, almond milk, chia seeds, and honey or maple syrup (if using) in a blender.
2. Blend until smooth and creamy.
3. If desired, add ice cubes to the blender and blend again until smooth.
4. Pour the Berry and Beet Detox Smoothie into a glass and serve immediately.
5. Garnish with additional berries or a sprinkle of chia seeds, if desired.
6. Enjoy this refreshing and nutritious smoothie as a healthy way to start your day or as a post-workout snack!

Nutritional Value (Approx.): Calories: 150 | Protein: 10g | Fat: 4g | Carbohydrates: 20g | Fiber: 6g

Citrus and Ginger Infused Water

Prep Time: 5 minutes | **Total Time**: 5 minutes | **Servings**: 1

Ingredients:

- 1/2 lemon, sliced
- 1/2 lime, sliced
- 1/2 orange, sliced
- 2-3 slices of fresh ginger
- 2 cups water
- Ice cubes (optional)
- Fresh mint leaves for garnish (optional)

Instructions:

1. Place lemon slices, lime slices, orange slices, and fresh ginger slices in a pitcher or glass.
2. Fill the pitcher or glass with water.
3. Let the Citrus and Ginger Infused Water sit for at least 30 minutes to allow the flavors to infuse.
4. If desired, add ice cubes to the glass before serving.
5. Garnish with fresh mint leaves for an extra burst of flavor and aroma.
6. Enjoy this refreshing and hydrating infused water as a delicious alternative to plain water throughout the day.

Nutritional Value (Approx.): Calories: 0 | Protein: 0g | Fat: 0g | Carbohydrates: 0g | Fiber: 0g

Probiotic Kefir Smoothie

Prep Time: 5 minutes | **Total Time**: 5 minutes | **Servings**: 1

Ingredients:

- 1/2 cup plain kefir
- 1/2 cup mixed berries (such as strawberries, blueberries, raspberries)
- 1/2 ripe banana
- 1 tablespoon honey or maple syrup (optional)
- 1/2 teaspoon vanilla extract
- Ice cubes (optional)

Instructions:

1. In a blender, combine plain kefir, mixed berries, ripe banana, honey or maple syrup (if using), and vanilla extract.
2. Blend until smooth and creamy.
3. If desired, add ice cubes to the blender and blend again until smooth.
4. Pour the Probiotic Kefir Smoothie into a glass and serve immediately.
5. Garnish with a few additional berries or a drizzle of honey, if desired.
6. Enjoy this delicious and gut-friendly smoothie as a nutritious snack or breakfast option!

Nutritional Value (Approx.): Calories: 200 | Protein: 6g | Fat: 3g | Carbohydrates: 40g | Fiber: 5g

Green Tea and Citrus Cooler

Prep Time: 5 minutes | **Cook Time**: 5 minutes | **Total Time**: 10 minutes | **Servings**: 2

Ingredients:

- 2 green tea bags
- 2 cups hot water
- 1/2 lemon, thinly sliced
- 1/2 lime, thinly sliced
- Ice cubes
- Fresh mint leaves for garnish (optional)

Instructions:

1. Place green tea bags in a teapot or heatproof pitcher.
2. Pour hot water over the tea bags and let steep for 3-5 minutes, depending on desired strength.
3. Remove the tea bags and allow the brewed tea to cool to room temperature.
4. Once cooled, transfer the tea to a refrigerator to chill for at least 1 hour.
5. In serving glasses, add a few slices of lemon and lime.
6. Pour the chilled green tea over the citrus slices.
7. Add ice cubes to each glass.
8. Garnish with fresh mint leaves, if desired.
9. Stir before drinking and enjoy this refreshing Green Tea and Citrus Cooler!

Nutritional Value (Approx.): Calories: 0 | Protein: 0g | Fat: 0g | Carbohydrates: 0g | Fiber: 0g

Immune-Boosting Ginger Lemon Tea

Prep Time: 5 minutes | **Cook Time**: 10 minutes | **Total Time**: 15 minutes | **Servings**: 2

Ingredients:

- 2 cups water
- 1-inch piece of fresh ginger, thinly sliced
- 1 lemon, juiced
- 2 tablespoons honey (or to taste)

Instructions:

1. In a small saucepan, bring water to a boil.
2. Add sliced ginger to the boiling water and reduce heat to low.
3. Simmer for 5-10 minutes to allow the ginger to infuse into the water.
4. Remove the saucepan from heat and strain out the ginger slices.
5. Stir in freshly squeezed lemon juice and honey to taste.
6. Pour the Immune-Boosting Ginger Lemon Tea into cups and serve hot.
7. Enjoy this soothing and immune-boosting tea as a comforting beverage during cold weather or when feeling under the weather.

Nutritional Value (Approx.): Calories: 60 | Protein: 0g | Fat: 0g | Carbohydrates: 17g | Fiber: 0g

Hydrating Cucumber Mint Water

Prep Time: 5 minutes | **Total Time**: 5 minutes | **Servings**: 2

Ingredients:

- 4 cups water
- 1/2 cucumber, thinly sliced
- Handful of fresh mint leaves
- Ice cubes

Instructions:

1. In a pitcher, combine water, thinly sliced cucumber, and fresh mint leaves.
2. Refrigerate the pitcher for at least 1 hour to allow the flavors to infuse.
3. When ready to serve, fill glasses with ice cubes.
4. Pour the Hydrating Cucumber Mint Water into the glasses.
5. Stir before drinking to distribute the flavors.
6. Enjoy this refreshing and hydrating beverage as a healthy alternative to sugary drinks!

Nutritional Value (Approx.): Calories: 0 | Protein: 0g | Fat: 0g | Carbohydrates: 0g | Fiber: 0g

Chapter Eight:

Sides and Small Plates

Roasted Brussels Sprouts with Balsamic Glaze

Prep Time: 10 minutes | **Cook Time**: 25 minutes | **Total Time**: 35 minutes | **Servings**: 4

Ingredients:

- 1 lb Brussels sprouts, trimmed and halved

- 2 tablespoons olive oil

- Salt and black pepper to taste

- 2 tablespoons balsamic glaze (store-bought or homemade)

Instructions:

1. Preheat the oven to 400°F (200°C) and line a baking sheet with parchment paper.

2. In a large bowl, toss Brussels sprouts with olive oil, salt, and black pepper until evenly coated.

3. Spread the Brussels sprouts in a single layer on the prepared baking sheet.

4. Roast in the preheated oven for 20-25 minutes, or until the Brussels sprouts are tender and caramelized, stirring halfway through.

5. Remove from the oven and drizzle with balsamic glaze.

6. Toss gently to coat the Brussels sprouts with the glaze.

7. Transfer to a serving dish and serve immediately.

8. Enjoy these delicious Roasted Brussels Sprouts with Balsamic Glaze as a flavorful side dish!

Nutritional Value (Approx.): Calories: 120 | Protein: 4g | Fat: 7g | Carbohydrates: 14g | Fiber: 4g

Sweet Potato and Kale Hash

Prep Time: 10 minutes | **Cook Time**: 20 minutes | **Total Time**: 30 minutes | **Servings**: 4

Ingredients:

- 2 large sweet potatoes, peeled and diced
- 1 tablespoon olive oil
- 1 small onion, diced
- 2 cloves garlic, minced
- 2 cups chopped kale leaves
- Salt and black pepper to taste

Instructions:

1. In a large skillet, heat olive oil over medium heat.
2. Add diced sweet potatoes to the skillet and cook for 8-10 minutes, stirring occasionally, until golden and tender.
3. Add diced onion and minced garlic to the skillet and cook for an additional 2-3 minutes, until the onion is translucent and fragrant.
4. Stir in chopped kale leaves and cook for 2-3 minutes, or until the kale is wilted.
5. Season with salt and black pepper to taste.
6. Remove from heat and transfer the Sweet Potato and Kale Hash to a serving dish.
7. Serve hot as a nutritious and hearty side dish or breakfast option.
8. Enjoy the flavorful combination of sweet potatoes and kale in this delicious hash!

Nutritional Value (Approx.): Calories: 180 | Protein: 3g | Fat: 4g | Carbohydrates: 35g | Fiber: 6g

Tomato and Avocado Salsa

Prep Time: 10 minutes | **Total Time**: 10 minutes | **Servings**: 4

Ingredients:

- 2 ripe tomatoes, diced
- 1 ripe avocado, diced
- 1/4 cup red onion, finely chopped
- 1/4 cup fresh cilantro, chopped
- 1 jalapeño pepper, seeded and finely chopped
- Juice of 1 lime
- Salt and black pepper to taste

Instructions:

1. In a medium bowl, combine diced tomatoes, diced avocado, finely chopped red onion, chopped cilantro, and finely chopped jalapeño pepper.
2. Squeeze fresh lime juice over the salsa.
3. Season with salt and black pepper to taste.
4. Gently toss all **Ingredients** until well combined.
5. Taste and adjust seasoning, if necessary.
6. Serve immediately as a topping for tacos, grilled meats, or as a dip with tortilla chips.
7. Enjoy the fresh and vibrant flavors of this Tomato and Avocado Salsa!

Nutritional Value (Approx.): Calories: 80 | Protein: 2g | Fat: 6g | Carbohydrates: 8g | Fiber: 4g

Garlic Sautéed Spinach

Prep Time: 5 minutes | **Cook Time**: 5 minutes | **Total Time**: 10 minutes | **Servings**: 4

Ingredients:

- 1 lb fresh spinach leaves
- 2 tablespoons olive oil
- 3 cloves garlic, minced
- Salt and black pepper to taste
- Pinch of red pepper flakes (optional)

Instructions:

1. Heat olive oil in a large skillet over medium heat.
2. Add minced garlic to the skillet and cook for 1-2 minutes, until fragrant.
3. Add fresh spinach leaves to the skillet in batches, stirring constantly, until wilted.
4. Season with salt, black pepper, and a pinch of red pepper flakes (if using).
5. Continue to cook for another 2-3 minutes, or until the spinach is tender and any excess liquid has evaporated.
6. Remove from heat and transfer the Garlic Sautéed Spinach to a serving dish.
7. Serve hot as a nutritious side dish or add it to omelets, pasta, or sandwiches.
8. Enjoy the simple yet flavorful taste of this Garlic Sautéed Spinach!

Nutritional Value (Approx.): Calories: 70 | Protein: 4g | Fat: 5g | Carbohydrates: 3g | Fiber: 2g

Fermented Veggie Slaw

Prep Time: 15 minutes | **Fermentation Time**: 3-5 days | **Total Time**: 3-5 days | **Servings**: 8

Ingredients:

- 4 cups shredded cabbage
- 2 carrots, grated
- 1 red bell pepper, thinly sliced
- 1 green bell pepper, thinly sliced
- 1/2 onion, thinly sliced
- 2 cloves garlic, minced
- 2 tablespoons sea salt
- 1 tablespoon whole mustard seeds
- 1 tablespoon grated ginger
- 1 teaspoon red pepper flakes (optional)
- Filtered water, as needed

Instructions:

1. In a large mixing bowl, combine shredded cabbage, grated carrots, sliced bell peppers, sliced onion, minced garlic, sea salt, mustard seeds, grated ginger, and red pepper flakes (if using).

2. Massage the vegetables with clean hands for 5-10 minutes, or until they start to release their juices.

3. Pack the vegetable mixture tightly into a clean glass jar, pressing down firmly to remove any air pockets.

4. Add filtered water if needed to ensure the vegetables are fully submerged.

5. Place a weight on top of the vegetables to keep them submerged under the brine.

6. Cover the jar loosely with a clean kitchen towel or cloth.

7. Allow the Fermented Veggie Slaw to ferment at room temperature for 3-5 days, depending on desired level of fermentation.

8. Check the slaw daily and press down on the weight to keep the vegetables submerged.

9. Once the desired level of fermentation is reached, transfer the jar to the refrigerator to slow down the fermentation process.

10. Enjoy the tangy and probiotic-rich Fermented Veggie Slaw as a tasty side dish or topping for sandwiches and salads!

Nutritional Value (Approx.): Calories: 30 | Protein: 1g | Fat: 0g | Carbohydrates: 7g | Fiber: 3g

Fermented Kimchi

Prep Time: 30 minutes | **Fermentation Time**: 3-7 days | **Total Time**: 3-7 days | **Servings**: 10

Ingredients:

- 1 medium Napa cabbage
- 1 daikon radish, julienned
- 4-6 green onions, chopped
- 3 cloves garlic, minced
- 1 tablespoon grated ginger
- 2 tablespoons Korean red pepper flakes (gochugaru)
- 2 tablespoons fish sauce or soy sauce
- 1 tablespoon sea salt
- Filtered water, as needed

Instructions:

1. Cut the Napa cabbage into quarters lengthwise and remove the core. Slice the cabbage crosswise into thin strips.

2. In a large mixing bowl, combine the sliced Napa cabbage, julienned daikon radish, chopped green onions, minced garlic, grated ginger, Korean red pepper flakes, fish sauce or soy sauce, and sea salt.

3. Massage the **Ingredients** together with clean hands for 5-10 minutes, or until the cabbage starts to soften and release its juices.

4. Pack the kimchi mixture tightly into clean glass jars, pressing down firmly to remove any air pockets.

5. Add filtered water if needed to ensure the vegetables are fully submerged.

6. Place a weight on top of the vegetables to keep them submerged under the brine.

7. Cover the jars loosely with clean kitchen towels or cloths.

8. Allow the Fermented Kimchi to ferment at room temperature for 3-7 days, depending on desired level of fermentation and temperature.

9. Check the kimchi daily and press down on the weight to keep the vegetables submerged.

10. Once the desired level of fermentation is reached, transfer the jars to the refrigerator to slow down the fermentation process.

11. Enjoy the spicy and tangy Fermented Kimchi as a flavorful condiment or side dish!

Nutritional Value (Approx.): Calories: 15 | Protein: 1g | Fat: 0g | Carbohydrates: 3g | Fiber: 1g

Cucumber and Mint Infused Water

Prep Time: 5 minutes | **Total Time**: 5 minutes | **Servings**: 2

Ingredients:

- 1/2 cucumber, thinly sliced
- Handful of fresh mint leaves
- 4 cups water
- Ice cubes

Instructions:

1. In a pitcher, combine thinly sliced cucumber and fresh mint leaves.

2. Add 4 cups of water to the pitcher.

3. Stir gently to combine the **Ingredients**.

4. Refrigerate the infused water for at least 1 hour to allow the flavors to meld.

5. When ready to serve, fill glasses with ice cubes.

6. Pour the Cucumber and Mint Infused Water into the glasses.

7. Garnish with additional cucumber slices and mint leaves, if desired.

8. Enjoy this refreshing and hydrating beverage as a delicious alternative to plain water!

Nutritional Value (Approx.): Calories: 0 | Protein: 0g | Fat: 0g | Carbohydrates: 0g | Fiber: 0g

Walnut and Spinach Pesto

Prep Time: 10 minutes | **Total Time**: 10 minutes | **Servings**: 6

Ingredients:

- 2 cups fresh spinach leaves
- 1/2 cup walnuts
- 2 cloves garlic
- 1/4 cup grated Parmesan cheese (or nutritional yeast for a vegan option)
- 1/4 cup olive oil
- Juice of 1 lemon
- Salt and black pepper to taste

Instructions:

1. In a food processor, combine fresh spinach leaves, walnuts, garlic, grated Parmesan cheese, olive oil, and lemon juice.
2. Pulse until the mixture forms a coarse paste, scraping down the sides of the bowl as needed.
3. Season with salt and black pepper to taste.
4. If the pesto is too thick, add more olive oil until desired consistency is reached.
5. Transfer the Walnut and Spinach Pesto to a jar or airtight container.
6. Store in the refrigerator for up to one week or use immediately as a flavorful topping or sauce for pasta, sandwiches, or salads.

Nutritional Value (Approx.): Calories: 160 | Protein: 4g | Fat: 15g | Carbohydrates: 4g | Fiber: 2g

Berries and Yogurt Parfait

Prep Time: 5 minutes | **Total Time**: 5 minutes | **Servings**: 1

Ingredients:

- 1/2 cup Greek yogurt
- 1/4 cup mixed berries (such as strawberries, blueberries, raspberries)
- 2 tablespoons granola
- 1 teaspoon honey (optional)
- Fresh mint leaves for garnish (optional)

Instructions:

1. In a serving glass or bowl, layer Greek yogurt, mixed berries, and granola.
2. Repeat the layers until the glass or bowl is filled.
3. Drizzle with honey, if desired, for added sweetness.
4. Garnish with fresh mint leaves, if using.
5. Serve immediately and enjoy this delicious and nutritious Berries and Yogurt Parfait as a breakfast, snack, or dessert option!

Nutritional Value (Approx.): Calories: 200 | Protein: 15g | Fat: 5g | Carbohydrates: 25g | Fiber: 5g

Mushroom and Garlic Stir-Fry

Prep Time: 10 minutes | **Cook Time**: 10 minutes | **Total Time**: 20 minutes | **Servings**: 2

Ingredients:

- 2 cups sliced mushrooms (such as button or cremini)
- 2 tablespoons olive oil
- 3 cloves garlic, minced
- 1 tablespoon soy sauce or tamari
- 1 teaspoon sesame oil
- 1 teaspoon rice vinegar
- Salt and black pepper to taste
- Fresh parsley for garnish (optional)

Instructions:

1. Heat olive oil in a large skillet or wok over medium-high heat.
2. Add minced garlic to the skillet and sauté for 1 minute, until fragrant.
3. Add sliced mushrooms to the skillet and cook for 5-7 minutes, stirring occasionally, until the mushrooms are tender and golden brown.
4. Stir in soy sauce or tamari, sesame oil, and rice vinegar.
5. Season with salt and black pepper to taste.
6. Continue to cook for another 2-3 minutes, allowing the flavors to meld.
7. Remove from heat and transfer the Mushroom and Garlic Stir-Fry to a serving dish.
8. Garnish with fresh parsley, if desired.
9. Serve hot as a savory side dish or add it to rice or noodles for a complete meal.
10. Enjoy the rich umami flavor of this Mushroom and Garlic Stir-Fry!

Nutritional Value (Approx.): Calories: 150 | Protein: 5g | Fat: 12g | Carbohydrates: 7g | Fiber: 2g

Chapter Nine:

Meal Planning and Tips

We'll explore the importance of meal planning and provide you with practical tips to streamline your meal preparation process, ensuring that you can maintain a healthy and balanced diet effortlessly.

Why Meal Planning Matters

- **Saves Time:** Planning your meals in advance saves time during busy weekdays, preventing last-minute stress and allowing you to focus on other tasks.

- **Promotes Healthy Eating:** Meal planning enables you to make healthier food choices by incorporating a variety of nutritious ingredients into your meals.

- **Reduces Food Waste:** By planning your meals, you can minimize food waste by buying only what you need and utilizing leftover ingredients efficiently.

- **Saves Money:** Planning your meals helps you stick to a budget by avoiding impulse purchases and reducing the frequency of eating out.

Tips for Effective Meal Planning

1. **Set Aside Time Weekly:** Dedicate a specific day each week to plan your meals for the upcoming week. This could be during the weekend or any other convenient time.

2. **Create a Menu:** Start by creating a weekly menu that includes breakfast, lunch, dinner, and snacks. Consider incorporating a variety of proteins, vegetables, fruits, whole grains, and healthy fats.

3. **Check Pantry and Fridge:** Before making your grocery list, take inventory of what you already have in your pantry and fridge. This prevents unnecessary purchases and ensures you use up perishable items.

4. **Plan Balanced Meals:** Aim for balanced meals that include a source of protein, healthy carbohydrates, and vegetables. Experiment with different cuisines and flavors to keep meals exciting.

5. **Prep Ingredients in Advance:** Save time during the week by prepping ingredients in advance, such as chopping vegetables, marinating proteins, or cooking grains.

6. **Batch Cooking:** Consider batch cooking certain components of meals, such as grains, proteins, or sauces, to have on hand for quick and easy assembly during busy days.

7. **Use Leftovers Creatively:** Embrace leftovers and repurpose them into new meals to prevent food waste. For example, leftover roasted vegetables can be added to salads or turned into a frittata.

8. **Stay Flexible:** Be flexible with your meal plan and allow room for adjustments based on changes in schedule or preferences. Don't be afraid to swap out planned meals if needed.

9. **Try New Recipes:** Use meal planning as an opportunity to try new recipes and experiment with different ingredients and cooking techniques.

10. **Enjoy the Process:** Meal planning should be enjoyable and empowering. Get creative in the kitchen, involve family members in the decision-making process, and savor the satisfaction of nourishing yourself and your loved ones.

30-Day Meal Plans for Optimal Health

Week 1

Day 1:

- Breakfast: Green Revitalizer Smoothie
- Lunch: Quinoa and Broccoli Salad with Citrus Dressing
- Dinner: Garlic Shrimp and Broccoli Stir-Fry

Day 2:

- Breakfast: Berry and Yogurt Parfait
- Lunch: Mediterranean Chickpea Salad
- Dinner: Spicy Black Bean Soup

Day 3:

- Breakfast: Mushroom and Spinach Omelette
- Lunch: Lentil and Sweet Potato Curry
- Dinner: Grilled Chicken and Kale Caesar Salad

Day 4:

- Breakfast: Matcha Green Tea Energy Balls
- Lunch: Mediterranean-Style Tuna with Olives
- Dinner: Tofu Stir-Fry with Ginger and Broccoli

Day 5:

- Breakfast: Avocado Toast with Tomatoes and Basil
- Lunch: Quinoa and Broccoli Salad with Citrus Dressing (leftovers)
- Dinner: Garlic Sautéed Spinach and Baked Salmon

Day 6:

- Breakfast: Oatmeal with Berries and Almonds
- Lunch: Stuffed Bell Peppers with Quinoa and Spinach
- Dinner: Turmeric Chicken with Roasted Vegetables

Day 7:

- Breakfast: Walnut and Spinach Pesto on Whole Grain Toast

- Lunch: Tomato-Basil White Bean and Quinoa Salad

- Dinner: Lentil and Mushroom Stew

Week 2

Day 8:

- Breakfast: Green Tea and Citrus Cooler

- Lunch: Quinoa and Broccoli Salad with Citrus Dressing (leftovers)

- Dinner: Spicy Turmeric Chicken with Sweet Potatoes (leftovers)

Day 9:

- Breakfast: Mixed Berry Smoothie Bowl

- Lunch: Mediterranean Chickpea Salad (leftovers)

- Dinner: Mushroom and Barley Risotto

Day 10:

- Breakfast: Chia Seed Pudding with Pomegranate

- Lunch: Roasted Chickpeas with Spices

- Dinner: Grilled Chicken and Kale Caesar Salad (leftovers)

Day 11:

- Breakfast: Turmeric Golden Milk Latte

- Lunch: Quinoa and Broccoli Salad with Citrus Dressing (leftovers)

- Dinner: Eggplant Salad with Walnuts and Mint

Day 12:

- Breakfast: Fluffy Sourdough Pancakes

- Lunch: Quinoa and Broccoli Salad with Citrus Dressing (leftovers)

- Dinner: Mediterranean Stuffed Peppers

Day 13:

- Breakfast: Pomegranate Yogurt Parfait

- Lunch: Lentil and Mushroom Stew (leftovers)

- Dinner: Garlic Shrimp and Broccoli Stir-Fry (leftovers)

Day 14:

- Breakfast: Matcha Green Tea Energy Balls
- Lunch: Tomato and Avocado Salsa with Whole Grain Tortilla Chips
- Dinner: Tofu Stir-Fry with Ginger and Broccoli (leftovers)

Week 3

Day 15:

- Breakfast: Green Revitalizer Smoothie
- Lunch: Mediterranean Chickpea Salad (leftovers)
- Dinner: Spicy Black Bean Soup (leftovers)

Day 16:

- Breakfast: Mixed Berry Smoothie Bowl
- Lunch: Lentil and Mushroom Stew (leftovers)
- Dinner: Mushroom and Barley Risotto (leftovers)

Day 17:

- Breakfast: Chia Seed Pudding with Pomegranate
- Lunch: Quinoa and Broccoli Salad with Citrus Dressing (leftovers)
- Dinner: Garlic Shrimp and Broccoli Stir-Fry (leftovers)

Day 18:

- Breakfast: Turmeric Golden Milk Latte
- Lunch: Mediterranean Stuffed Peppers (leftovers)
- Dinner: Eggplant Salad with Walnuts and Mint (leftovers)

Day 19:

- Breakfast: Fluffy Sourdough Pancakes
- Lunch: Tomato and Avocado Salsa with Whole Grain Tortilla Chips
- Dinner: Tofu Stir-Fry with Ginger and Broccoli (leftovers)

Day 20:

- Breakfast: Pomegranate Yogurt Parfait
- Lunch: Roasted Chickpeas with Spices
- Dinner: Grilled Chicken and Kale Caesar Salad (leftovers)

Day 21:

- Breakfast: Matcha Green Tea Energy Balls
- Lunch: Quinoa and Broccoli Salad with Citrus Dressing (leftovers)
- Dinner: Spicy Turmeric Chicken with Sweet Potatoes (leftovers)

Week 4

Day 22:

- Breakfast: Green Revitalizer Smoothie
- Lunch: Mediterranean Chickpea Salad (leftovers)
- Dinner: Garlic Shrimp and Broccoli Stir-Fry (leftovers)

Day 23:

- Breakfast: Mixed Berry Smoothie Bowl
- Lunch: Lentil and Mushroom Stew (leftovers)
- Dinner: Mushroom and Barley Risotto (leftovers)

Day 24:

- Breakfast: Chia Seed Pudding with Pomegranate
- Lunch: Quinoa and Broccoli Salad with Citrus Dressing (leftovers)
- Dinner: Mediterranean Stuffed Peppers (leftovers)

Day 25:

- Breakfast: Turmeric Golden Milk Latte
- Lunch: Tomato and Avocado Salsa with Whole Grain Tortilla Chips
- Dinner: Tofu Stir-Fry with Ginger and Broccoli (leftovers)

Day 26:

- Breakfast: Fluffy Sourdough Pancakes
- Lunch: Roasted Chickpeas with Spices
- Dinner: Grilled Chicken and Kale Caesar Salad (leftovers)

Day 27:

- Breakfast: Pomegranate Yogurt Parfait
- Lunch: Quinoa and Broccoli Salad with Citrus Dressing (leftovers)

* Dinner: Spicy Black Bean Soup (leftovers)

Day 28:

* Breakfast: Matcha Green Tea Energy Balls

* Lunch: Mediterranean Chickpea Salad (leftovers)

* Dinner: Eggplant Salad with Walnuts and Mint (leftovers)

Day 29:

* Breakfast: Green Revitalizer Smoothie

* Lunch: Lentil and Mushroom Stew (leftovers)

* Dinner: Spicy Turmeric Chicken with Sweet Potatoes (leftovers)

Day 30:

* Breakfast: Mixed Berry Smoothie Bowl

* Lunch: Quinoa and Broccoli Salad with Citrus Dressing (leftovers)

* Dinner: Mushroom and Barley Risotto (leftovers)

Shopping Lists for Health-Promoting Foods

Week 1:

- **Proteins:**
    - Chicken breast
    - Shrimp
    - Tofu
    - Eggs
- **Vegetables:**
    - Spinach
    - Broccoli
    - Kale
    - Bell peppers
    - Mushrooms
    - Garlic
    - Onion
- **Fruits:**
    - Green apple
    - Lemon
    - Berries (strawberries, blueberries, raspberries)
    - Avocado
    - Tomato
- **Grains/Legumes:**
    - Quinoa
    - Lentils
    - Barley
    - Black beans
    - Chickpeas
- **Dairy/Alternatives:**

- Greek yogurt
  - Almond milk
- **Pantry Staples:**
  - Chia seeds
  - Olive oil
  - Soy sauce or tamari
  - Sesame oil
  - Rice vinegar
  - Spices (turmeric, garlic powder, black pepper, red pepper flakes)

Week 2:

- **Proteins:**
  - Salmon fillets
  - Tuna
  - Eggs
- **Vegetables:**
  - Cucumber
  - Bell peppers
  - Mushrooms
  - Garlic
  - Onion
  - Eggplant
- **Fruits:**
  - Berries (blueberries, raspberries)
  - Pomegranate
  - Lemon
- **Grains/Legumes:**
  - Whole grain bread
  - Brown rice

- Whole grain tortilla chips
- **Dairy/Alternatives:**
  - Greek yogurt
- **Pantry Staples:**
  - Walnuts
  - Parmesan cheese
  - Honey
  - Turmeric powder
  - Fish sauce
  - Nutritional yeast (for vegan option)
  - Whole grain tortilla chips

Week 3:

- **Proteins:**
  - Chicken breast
  - Tofu
  - Eggs
- **Vegetables:**
  - Spinach
  - Broccoli
  - Mushrooms
  - Garlic
  - Onion
- **Fruits:**
  - Mixed berries
  - Pomegranate
  - Lemon
- **Grains/Legumes:**
  - Oats

- Chickpeas
  - Quinoa
- **Dairy/Alternatives:**
  - Greek yogurt
  - Almond milk
- **Pantry Staples:**
  - Chia seeds
  - Olive oil
  - Soy sauce or tamari
  - Sesame oil
  - Rice vinegar
  - Spices (cinnamon, ginger, garlic powder, black pepper)

Week 4:

- **Proteins:**
  - Shrimp
  - Tuna
  - Eggs
- **Vegetables:**
  - Brussels sprouts
  - Sweet potato
  - Spinach
  - Mushrooms
  - Garlic
  - Onion
- **Fruits:**
  - Berries (raspberries, strawberries)
  - Avocado
- **Grains/Legumes:**

- Quinoa
  - Lentils
- **Dairy/Alternatives:**
  - Greek yogurt
- **Pantry Staples:**
  - Olive oil
  - Garlic powder
  - Black pepper
  - Red pepper flakes
  - Balsamic glaze

Recommended Kitchen Tools and Gadgets

Preparing health-promoting meals becomes easier and more enjoyable with the right kitchen tools and gadgets. Here's a list of recommended items to equip your kitchen:

1. **High-Speed Blender:** Ideal for making smoothies, soups, sauces, and homemade nut milk. Look for one with multiple speed settings and a powerful motor.

2. **Food Processor:** Perfect for chopping, slicing, shredding, and pureeing ingredients. Useful for making homemade dips, sauces, and energy balls.

3. **Vegetable Spiralizer:** Great for creating vegetable noodles from zucchini, carrots, and other veggies. A fun way to incorporate more vegetables into your diet.

4. **Steamer Basket:** Essential for steaming vegetables while preserving their nutrients and flavors. Can also be used to steam fish and dumplings.

5. **Salad Spinner:** Makes washing and drying salad greens quick and efficient. Ensures crisp and dry lettuce leaves for salads.

6. **Mandoline Slicer:** Provides uniform slices of fruits and vegetables with ease. Useful for making salads, gratins, and garnishes.

7. **Immersion Blender:** Convenient for blending soups and sauces directly in the pot. Offers easy cleanup compared to traditional blenders.

8. **Cast Iron Skillet:** Versatile and durable cookware for sautéing, searing, and baking. Provides even heat distribution and adds trace amounts of iron to your food.

9. **Non-Stick Cookware Set:** Includes pots and pans with a non-stick coating for low-fat cooking and easy cleanup. Choose PFOA-free options for health-conscious cooking.

10. **Food Scale:** Helps accurately measure ingredients for portion control and precise baking. Essential for following recipes and tracking food intake.

11. **Microplane Grater/Zester:** Ideal for grating citrus zest, ginger, garlic, and hard cheeses. Adds intense flavor to dishes with minimal effort.

12. **Kitchen Knife Set:** Invest in a high-quality knife set with a chef's knife, utility knife, and paring knife. Sharp knives make food prep safer and more efficient.

13. **Baking Sheet and Wire Rack:** Essential for roasting vegetables, baking cookies, and cooling baked goods. Opt for heavy-duty, non-toxic materials.

14. **Instant-Read Thermometer:** Ensures meats, poultry, and fish are cooked to the correct internal temperature for food safety.

15. **Silicone Baking Mats:** Reusable alternatives to parchment paper for non-stick baking. Environmentally friendly and easy to clean.

16. **Vegetable Steamer:** Offers a healthy cooking method by preserving nutrients in vegetables. Fits inside pots of various sizes for versatility.

17. **Herb Scissors:** Streamline the process of chopping fresh herbs for garnishes, salads, and marinades. Features multiple blades for efficient cutting.

CONCLUSION

Incorporating health-promoting foods into your daily diet can profoundly impact your overall well-being and longevity. By understanding the science behind these foods and their benefits, you empower yourself to make informed dietary choices that support your body's natural defense systems.

"Eat to Beat Disease: The New Science of How Your Body Can Heal Itself," revolutionizes the way we think about food and its role in our health, which presents a comprehensive guide to using food as a powerful tool to combat disease and promote wellness. This book synthesizes cutting-edge research and practical advice, offering a roadmap to harnessing the body's innate healing capabilities through diet.

The concept is that our bodies are equipped with five key defense systems that work synergistically to protect and maintain health: angiogenesis, regeneration, the microbiome, DNA protection, and immunity. By understanding and supporting these systems, we can optimize our health and reduce the risk of chronic diseases.

1. Angiogenesis: This process involves the growth of new blood vessels, which is crucial for healing wounds, preventing cancer, and supporting cardiovascular health. Dr. Li explains how certain foods, such as berries, citrus fruits, and leafy greens, contain bioactive compounds that promote healthy angiogenesis, while others, like processed meats and high-sugar foods, can disrupt this delicate balance.

2. Regeneration: The body's ability to regenerate and repair itself is vital for maintaining health and vitality. Stem cells play a key role in this process. Foods like dark chocolate, red wine, and certain teas contain compounds that stimulate stem cell activity, aiding in tissue repair and renewal. Also emphasizes the importance of a diet rich in these regenerative foods to support the body's natural healing processes.

3. Microbiome: The trillions of microorganisms living in our gut influence digestion, immunity, and even mental health. A diverse and balanced microbiome is essential for overall well-being, highlights the benefits of fermented foods, such as yogurt, kefir, and kimchi, which introduce beneficial bacteria into the gut. Fiber-rich foods, like fruits, vegetables, and whole grains, also nourish the microbiome, fostering a healthy digestive environment.

4. DNA Protection: Our DNA is constantly under attack from environmental factors and oxidative stress. Antioxidants and other protective compounds found in foods like berries, nuts, and cruciferous vegetables help safeguard our genetic material. It discusses how these foods can prevent mutations and reduce the risk of diseases like cancer.

5. Immunity: A robust immune system is essential for defending against infections and chronic diseases. Nutrient-dense foods, such as citrus fruits, garlic, and ginger, can boost immune function. It provides practical tips on incorporating these immune-boosting foods into daily meals to enhance the body's defenses.

The book also addresses the concept of **"food as medicine,"** illustrating how dietary choices can have a profound impact on health outcomes. He provides numerous examples of how specific foods can be used to prevent and even treat various conditions. For instance, he explains how tomatoes and their rich lycopene content can reduce the risk of prostate cancer, or how the sulforaphane in broccoli can help detoxify harmful substances in the body.

The book is filled with practical advice on integrating health-promoting foods into your diet which emphasizes the importance of variety and balance, encouraging readers to experiment with different foods and flavors. He provides a wealth of recipes and meal plans that make it easy to incorporate these principles into daily life.

Summary of Key Takeaways:

- **Variety is Crucial:** Embrace a diverse range of fruits, vegetables, nuts, seeds, whole grains, and legumes to ensure a broad spectrum of nutrients and bioactive compounds.

- **Incorporate Superfoods:** Foods like berries, leafy greens, nuts, seeds, and fermented foods should be staples in your diet due to their potent health benefits.

- **Balance Your Diet:** While focusing on health-promoting foods, maintain a balanced diet that includes all food groups in appropriate proportions.

- **Use Food to Target Specific Health Goals:** Understand which foods support your unique health needs, whether it's boosting immunity, protecting DNA, promoting angiogenesis, or fostering a healthy microbiome.

- **Practical Tips for Meal Planning:** Dr. Li provides actionable advice and meal planning strategies to help you seamlessly integrate these foods into your daily routine.

Practical Application:

This book is not just about theoretical knowledge; it provides practical steps to transform your diet and, consequently, your health. Here are some specific recommendations for incorporating his advice into your daily life:

- **Smoothies:** Start your day with a nutrient-packed smoothie that includes leafy greens, berries, chia seeds, and almond milk. This simple habit can significantly boost your intake of vitamins, minerals, and antioxidants.

- **Salads:** Make salads a daily staple. Include a variety of colorful vegetables, fruits, nuts, and seeds. Use olive oil-based dressings to add healthy fats and enhance nutrient absorption.

- **Snacks:** Replace processed snacks with healthful options like nuts, seeds, and fruit. Consider making your own trail mix or energy balls using ingredients like oats, honey, and superfood powders.

- **Fermented Foods:** Incorporate fermented foods into your diet regularly. Add a serving of yogurt or kefir to your breakfast, or enjoy kimchi or sauerkraut with your meals.

- **Balanced Meals:** Aim for balanced meals that include a source of protein, healthy fats, and a variety of vegetables. For example, a dinner of grilled salmon, quinoa, and a side of steamed broccoli provides a good mix of nutrients.

- **Hydration:** Don't forget the importance of staying hydrated. Drink plenty of water throughout the day and consider infusing it with slices of citrus fruits, cucumber, or herbs for added flavor and benefits.

Measurement Conversion

Understanding measurement conversions is essential when preparing recipes, especially if you're using a mix of sources from different regions. Here is a comprehensive guide to help you convert common cooking measurements:

Volume Conversions

Metric to US Standard:

- 1 milliliter (ml) = 0.034 fluid ounces (fl oz)
- 100 milliliters (ml) = 3.4 fluid ounces (fl oz)
- 240 milliliters (ml) = 1 cup (US)
- 500 milliliters (ml) = 2.1 cups (US)
- 1 liter (L) = 4.2 cups (US) = 33.8 fluid ounces (fl oz)

US Standard to Metric:

- 1 teaspoon (tsp) = 5 milliliters (ml)
- 1 tablespoon (tbsp) = 15 milliliters (ml)
- 1 fluid ounce (fl oz) = 30 milliliters (ml)
- 1 cup = 240 milliliters (ml)
- 1 pint (pt) = 480 milliliters (ml) = 0.48 liters (L)
- 1 quart (qt) = 960 milliliters (ml) = 0.96 liters (L)
- 1 gallon (gal) = 3.8 liters (L)

Weight Conversions

Metric to US Standard:

- 1 gram (g) = 0.035 ounces (oz)
- 100 grams (g) = 3.5 ounces (oz)
- 500 grams (g) = 17.6 ounces (oz) = 1.1 pounds (lb)
- 1 kilogram (kg) = 35.3 ounces (oz) = 2.2 pounds (lb)

US Standard to Metric:

- 1 ounce (oz) = 28 grams (g)
- 1 pound (lb) = 454 grams (g) = 0.454 kilograms (kg)

Temperature Conversions

Celsius to Fahrenheit:

- $°F = °C × 9/5 + 32$ $°F = °C × 9/5 + 32$

Fahrenheit to Celsius:

- $°C = (°F − 32) × 5/9$ $°C = (°F − 32) × 5/9$

Common Temperature Conversions:

- 180°C = 356°F
- 200°C = 392°F
- 220°C = 428°F
- 250°C = 482°F

Baking Conversions

Flour:

- 1 cup all-purpose flour = 120 grams
- 1 cup whole wheat flour = 130 grams

Sugar:

- 1 cup granulated sugar = 200 grams
- 1 cup powdered sugar = 120 grams
- 1 cup brown sugar = 220 grams

Butter:

- 1 cup butter = 227 grams = 2 sticks (US)

Common Ingredient Conversions

Liquids:

- 1 cup water = 240 milliliters (ml)
- 1 cup milk = 240 milliliters (ml)
- 1 tablespoon olive oil = 15 milliliters (ml)

Dry Ingredients:

- 1 cup oats = 90 grams
- 1 cup rice = 200 grams
- 1 cup dried beans = 180 grams

Useful Equivalents

- 1 tablespoon (tbsp) = 3 teaspoons (tsp)
- 1 cup = 16 tablespoons (tbsp)
- 1 pint (US) = 2 cups = 32 fluid ounces (fl oz)
- 1 quart (US) = 4 cups = 64 fluid ounces (fl oz)
- 1 gallon (US) = 16 cups = 128 fluid ounces (fl oz)